DR. ABRAVANEL'S BODY TYPE DIET AND LIFETIME NUTRITION PLAN

DR. ABRAVANEL'S BODY TYPE DIET AND LIFETIME NUTRITION PLAN

ELLIOT D. ABRAVANEL, M.D. AND ELIZABETH A. KING

ILLUSTRATIONS BY VIVIEN COHEN

BANTAM BOOKS
TORONTO · NEW YORK · LONDON · SYDNEY

This or any other diet should be followed only
under a doctor's supervision.

DR. ABRAVANEL'S BODY TYPE DIET
A Bantam Book / March 1983

Library of Congress Cataloging in Publication Data

Abravanel, Elliot D.
  Dr. Abravanel's Body type diet and lifetime
nutrition plan.

  1. Reducing diets—Recipes. 2. Reducing exercises.
3. Physiognomy. I. King, Elizabeth A. II. Title.
III. Title: Doctor Abravanel's Body type diet and
lifetime nutrition plan. IV. Title: Body type diet and
lifetime nutrition plan.
RM222.2.A25 1983   646.7'5   82-45942
ISBN 0-553-05036-2

  Published simultaneously in the United States and Canada

PRINTED IN THE UNITED STATES OF AMERICA

0 9 8 7 6 5

CONTENTS

FOREWORD

I live in Southern California, and it seems to me that nowhere is the connection between health and beauty more obvious than it is here. The intense light of the desert, the year-round warmth and perpetual sunshine invite a style of life that is lived largely out of doors. It is impossible for anyone to hide an unhealthy, out-of-shape body under layers of heavy, concealing clothing.

In my medical practice I see many intelligent, health-conscious people who are concerned about their weight. They want to look good, but they are well aware that good health is the key ingredient to true beauty. My Body Type Diet and Lifetime Nutrition Plan is designed with this kind of person in mind. This program is not just a way of losing weight, but an entirely new set of *principles of dieting,* based on the most modern theories of the biochemical interaction of foods with the body.

A diet should transform your body, not just change it in a superficial way. A body is not a static entity from which fat can be peeled away like layers of an onion. The transformation must come from within, for only a healthy, balanced body can maintain its ideal weight. Overweight itself indicates imbalance in the system. Defining exactly what imbalances exist, and then correcting them through diet *while you are losing weight* is precisely what the Body Type Diet and Lifetime Nutrition Plan accomplishes.

NO SINGLE DIET WORKS FOR EVERYONE

The most important principle of body type dieting, which I have evolved in the course of treating thousands of overweight patients, is that *there is no one diet that works for everyone, and there never will be.* Rather, there are four very different body types—that is, four types of metabolism—defined by which of the body's four major glands (the gonads, the adrenal glands, the thyroid glands, and the pituitary glands) is dominant in the system. Each of these four body types has its own, very specific dieting requirements.

DISCOVER WHICH OF THE FOUR BODY TYPES YOU ARE

The Body Type Diet has an essential preliminary step which no other diet has: the step of determining your body type. You'll learn how to do it in Chapter 5. Knowing your body type tells you a great deal about your overweight. It explains, first, how you became fat—which foods you felt irresistible cravings for, and ate too much of, in the past. It also explains how you look in an overweight condition—where you have fat deposits, and which parts of your body remain relatively slim despite your overweight.

Even more important, your body type determines your strategy for getting, and staying, slender. It determines which foods you must eliminate from your diet, even though other people just as overweight as you are can safely eat them and still lose weight. It determines which foods you *must* eat while dieting in order to free yourself from cravings and achieve metabolic balance. It even determines *when* you should eat—whether you will lose weight more easily by eating your biggest meal early, in the middle, or late in the day.

In short, your body type determines what type of diet will work for you. It provides you with a guide through the confusing muddle of diets available everywhere today, and lets you custom-tailor a weight loss program to fit *your* metabolic needs.

THE BODY TYPE DIET PROGRAM

Once you know your body type, you start on your Body Type Weight Loss Diet and follow it for a week. What happens after that depends on how much you want and need to lose. If you have only a few extra pounds, you change at this point to the Last Five

Pounds Diet for your body type. If you have more excess weight, you follow your Weight Loss Diet for up to three weeks before changing to the Last Five Pounds Diet for a week. This four-week program can then be repeated, if necessary, until you have reached your weight goal.

When you do reach your weight goal (and you will!), you move on to the Health and Weight Maintenance Diet for your body type. This is a flexible and easily followed eating program for a lifetime of good health at your ideal weight.

WHAT IS YOUR IDEAL WEIGHT?

Your ideal weight is not defined by tables or numbers. It is, very simply, the weight at which you look your best and feel wonderful. It is the weight at which you are free from "pockets" of fat and cellulite, at which your body is well proportioned and attractive. It is the weight at which you have abundant energy, both mental and physical, and at which you rest well and get full value from your rest.

A table of heights and weights cannot tell you what this weight is for you, because no table or chart has ever taken into account the fact that the ideal weight differs, among people of the same height, according to body type. You will see when we look at the four body types why the adrenal and gonadal types are always slightly heavier, at their ideal weight, than the thyroid or pituitary types. Because of this natural variation, the only way to be sure of determining your ideal weight is to reach it—through Body Type Dieting.

THE MOST EFFECTIVE WEIGHT LOSS DIET— AND THE BEST OF HEALTH

Modern medicine has a good idea of what sort of things shorten life. Obesity, smoking, poor diet, lack of exercise, lack of sufficient rest, and environmental pollution—all are contributors to shorter life expectancy. But it is still not entirely clear how long a person might live if all circumstances were completely right.

Some experts in genetics believe that our bodies are programmed to die after a certain number of years, or breaths, or heartbeats. Others believe that our lives are not limited by time alone, but by other factors which cause our systems to begin to decline. Some of these limiting factors are under our control and can be eliminated; wrong eating habits are certainly one factor that we can control.

The Body Type Diet and Lifetime Nutrition Plan is intended, ultimately, as a contribution towards slowing—and reversing—the body's decline. It is for weight loss, yes. My experience has shown me over and over again that the Body Type Diet produces the fastest, safest, and most effective weight loss for each of the body types. But it is also designed for improvement in the quality of life. My aim has been to help all who follow these diets make the most of their potential to enjoy life in all its fullness. After all, life is not just a salted cracker or a scoop of cottage cheese. It's a banquet.

Elliot D. Abravanel, M.D.
Los Angeles, California
September 1982

1

FINDING THE
RIGHT DIET
FOR YOU

Most people today believe that to be slim is necessarily to be healthy. They are mistaken; most diets are so unhealthy as to be useless in the long run. In fact, most diets aren't even useful in the short run, even for weight loss, because the weight lost invariably comes right back.

Occasionally, a diet will work for some lucky dieter. But for every dieter who loses weight, there are hundreds more who fail. And no one ever explains *why* a diet works, when it does, or why it fails.

The Body Type Diet answers these questions. Body Type Dieting is not just another peel-away-the-pounds fad. Rather, it is a systematic medical program relating different types of diet to different types of body, in order to enable each individual to find the diet that will be effective, safe and healthy for him.

HOW I DISCOVERED
THE IMPORTANCE OF
BODY TYPES

I developed the concept of the Body Type Diet and Lifetime Nutrition Plan in the context of my practice of family medicine. Unlike medical specialists, who focus their attention on one system of the body or another, I am a generalist, accustomed to looking at my patients as whole people in whom all parts of the body have to work together for health. Naturally one of the problems often presented to me is the problem of overweight, and I am often asked for advice about diet. Since the importance of maintaining one's ideal weight is, from a health standpoint, beyond dispute, I determined to find a way to help my patients achieve this goal.

But I was not fully satisfied with any of the diets available today. What struck me was that while one or two patients would lose weight on one or the other of the many popular diets that exist in the marketplace, most of them either failed to lose, or lost weight and quickly gained it back.

I decided to take a closer look at those of my patients who did lose weight successfully, and to isolate those factors which were the keys to success.

Two patients, who happened to come to my office on the same day, illustrated clearly what I discovered. The two were both women, good friends who had decided to diet together for mutual reinforcement. Both had managed to lose about nine pounds; one wanted to lose six more, the other sixteen more pounds. Both had been on a popular diet which was low in protein and fats and high in complex carbohydrates. But there the similarity ended.

The first patient, whom I will call Anna, was the one within six pounds of her weight goal, and she looked very well. She had lost her weight from the right places—her hips and thighs, rather than her face, which had never been fat. She told me that she felt healthy and vigorous even though she was dieting, and she looked that way too.

The second patient, Joanne, was a contrast to Anna in almost every way. She retained "pockets" of fat on her outer thighs which, she told me, she'd been unable to lose. Her face was gaunt and she had a pasty, unhealthy color. Moreover, she was having difficulty sticking to her diet, and was constantly suffering from an intense craving for sweets.

What was particularly interesting to me was that both women had followed exactly the same diet. I knew them both, and was confident that Joanne had not been "cheating"; she was highly motivated to lose weight. Obviously, the difference was not in the diet but in the dieter—or rather, in the *interaction* of dieter and diet. The way the diet worked for Anna was obviously not the way it worked for Joanne.

Examining the two women, I discovered that their bodies were indeed very different. Anna had a very steady, strong metabolism. She had excellent digestion, was active all day and had relatively little variation in her energy level. Joanne was a very different type; she was livelier than Anna, but more given to ups and downs in energy. She had intense nervous energy, but tended to "crash" in the late afternoon if she wasn't careful. She drank a lot of coffee and diet cola to keep herself going. In short, she was more highly-strung and more delicate than Anna.

I decided to put Joanne on a completely different diet from the high-carbohydrate one that had seemed to work for Anna. The diet I selected was high in protein, lower in carbohydrates, and eliminated all caffeine drinks. The idea of this diet was to provide a steadying balance for her delicate, highly-strung system. Meanwhile, I told Anna to continue as she had been, until she had lost the rest of her excess weight.

To my delight, Joanne responded beautifully to her changed program. After just a week on the diet she began to look healthier. Her face, which had been so gaunt, filled out and her cheeks were rosy. But more important to her, she began to lose the pockets of fat on her thighs. Within four weeks she had lost the entire sixteen pounds. Now, five years after that memorable month, she is still at her ideal weight.

Anna, meanwhile, continued on her high-carbohydrate diet and by the end of the next week she had lost her remaining six pounds. Now both women had dieted successfully—but on diets which, like their metabolisms, were diametrically different.

The conclusion reached from Joanne, Anna and thousands of other patients over the years is that success in dieting depends on the particular character of the dieter's metabolism. If this vital factor is not considered, the diet will inevitably fail. Without a system for determining what type of body a dieter has, dieters and their physicians alike are at the mercy of chance and guesswork.

THE FOUR BODY TYPES

Individuals process foods differently—this much is common knowledge. We have all observed that some people can eat much more than others without gaining weight. Also, some people need more of different kinds of food—more protein, more carbohydrates, or more fats. And some people are affected adversely by foods which other people tolerate well. These facts are indications of a vitally important truth: Each person has his or her body type based upon how food is metabolised in the body.

There are a number of traditional systems for classifying individuals according to body type. Perhaps the best known is the classification into *ectomorph* (the slim, rangy body type), *endomorph* (the rounder, plumper body type) or *mesomorph* (the thicker, more muscular body type). The limitation of this system is that it is purely descriptive; it doesn't tell *why* a person is slim, round or muscular.

Another system is that used in classical Chinese medicine, which classifies bodies according to which of the five "elements" (earth, water, fire, air or ether) predominates. While this system has a good deal of value and is useful in certain courses of treatment, I wanted to find one which would be both highly accurate and easier to use. I wanted a system that would *prescribe* the right diet while *describing* the body type.

I set about to develop such a system. I began to classify individuals according to which of their four major glands—the pituitary gland, the thyroid gland, the adrenal glands and the gonads or sex glands—was most active, or *dominant,* in their metabolism. According to this system, I could then classify a person as a "pituitary type, a "thyroid type," an "adrenal type" or a "gonadal type."

The inspiration for my system of body types came from Dr. Henry Bieler, the great physician and nutritionist and author of the book *Food Is Your Best Medicine.* Dr. Bieler shows in this book how it is possible to distinguish between individuls with a dominant thyroid and a dominant adrenal gland on the basis of fairly obvious physical characteristics. Dr. Bieler's "thyroid type" is slender, fine-boned, long-limbed—much like the classic ectomorph. His "adrenal type" is squarer in shape, thicker and more solid, and closely resembles the classic mesomorph. Bieler also suspected that there might be a third body type, the pituitary type, but he was not certain of this and did not fully define what this type would look like.

I took Dr. Bieler's original work as my point of departure. I went on to make a full description of the pituitary type. I also found that, while three types are sufficient to classify men, women require a fourth classification, which I named the "gonadal type."

I also realized that although Dr. Bieler's suggested system of body types was useful descriptively, he had not done any work relating the types to their best diet for weight loss. This was to be my task. I studied carefully the relationships between foods and the glands, and on this basis was able to develop, for each type, the precise diet to enable people with that body type to lose weight most effectively.

Once you know your own body type, you will know, first, what type of metabolism you have—that is, how quickly or slowly, efficiently or inefficiently, your body processes food. Second, you will know how your body reacts to each of the three classes of food: proteins, carbohydrates and fats. Third, you will know which foods within the three classes are most useful to your type of metabolism. Finally, you will know the characteristic weaknesses of your metabolism which must be offset by diet. On the basis of this information I will help you to select the precise Body Type Diet that will work for you.

It is important for you to realize that your Body Type Diet is *not* a crash diet which you will follow until you reach your desired weight, and then forget. *It is a lifetime eating program designed for improved health, energy and vitality at your ideal weight.*

For this reason I do not want you to follow your Body Type Diet blindly. I want you to really understand your body type, to see what your metabolic strengths are and what potential weaknesses you may have.

In the next chapters we are going to look at the Body Type Diet Program in detail. You will learn what body type you are, and you will see how your metabolism can be strengthened and balanced through the foods proper for *your* body type.

You will then be ready to take control of your health and your weight, and to use the tool of your Body Type Diet to create the ideal body *for you*.

2
THE BASIC FEATURES OF THE BODY TYPE DIET

There are certain basic rules for healthy, balanced dieting which apply to all of the body types, and which you must understand whether you turn out to be a gonadal, adrenal, thyroid or pituitary type. Understanding the rules you will encounter in this chapter will enable you to appreciate your own Body Type Diet more fully, and to follow it more intelligently.

RULE #1: WORK WITH YOUR BODY TYPE.

Each Body Type Diet is an individualized application of the same basic strategy: a strategy of utilizing foods that are in harmony with the metabolic needs of your body type. By using foods in this way it is possible to create a state of metabolic balance in which your body can reach and maintain its ideal weight.

For each of the four body types, the particular combination of foods is different; but in each case the *approach* to selecting foods is the same. The approach is, fundamentally, to *restrict* foods which are stimulating to the dominant gland of your body type (these are your body type's "danger foods"), and to *encourage* foods which strengthen and support your less-active glands. You'll discover in Chapter 3 precisely which foods perform these functions for your own body type, and how this approach works so effectively to enable you to reach your ideal weight.

RULE #2: FOLLOW THE BODY TYPE DIET SEQUENCE.

Each body type has a four-week sequence of diets, consisting of three weeks of the Body Type Weight Loss Diet and a fourth week on the Last Five Pounds Diet. This four-week sequence can be repeated as many times as necessary to reach your ideal weight.

If you have only a small amount of weight to lose, you may only need to follow a part of the four-week sequence. See your own Body Type Diet for details.

The Weight Loss Diet for each body type uses the strategy described in Rule #1 to produce fast, effective weight loss. The Last Five Pounds Diet takes the basic strategy one step further: it restricts your body type's "danger foods" still further, and provides special dieting helps which are used for this phase of the sequence only.

The purpose of the Last Five Pounds Diet is to help your body deal with the most stubborn of all dieting problems: the tendency of your body to reach "plateaus" in dieting, at which weight loss unaccountably slows or stops. I have found that it is possible to overcome the problem of plateaus by using a special diet every fourth week, the interval at which plateaus most often occur.

The diet is called the Last Five Pounds Diet to distinguish the most difficult of all plateaus, the one that occurs when you are down to your last five pounds of excess weight. As everyone who has dieted knows, these pounds are far harder to lose than the five, fifteen or fifty pounds that come before, because they are made up of a special kind of fat called "cellulite."

Cellulite is the wrinkly, "cottage cheese" fat that occurs on almost every woman, and some men, most often on the hips, thighs, abdomen and upper arms. The special strategies of the Last Five Pounds Diet are designed to facilitate the burning of cellulite, as well as to eliminate the plateaus that occur regularly during a weight loss program.

THE CALORIC LEVEL

Each Weight Loss Diet contains about 1200 calories per day, and each Last Five Pounds Diet about 1000 calories. Experience has convinced me that the 1200 calorie-per-day level is the safest, most effective one for long-term, permanent weight loss. Reducing calories below this level for any extended period runs the risk of nutritional deficiencies. However, a temporarily lower caloric intake can be used to break plateaus.

The caloric level is not the most important aspect of the diet, by any means. Reducing the number of calories consumed is a necessary ingredient in losing weight, but is not enough in itself to insure success. The laws of physics cannot be changed; you cannot lose weight unless you eat fewer calories than you burn up in activity. If you eat *more* calories than you burn up, you will gain weight. But the body is not a machine, requiring only energy to run. It is an organic system with many nutritional requirements, all of which must be met if you want the weight you lose to stay away.

BALANCE AND NUTRITIONAL SUFFICIENCY

The Body Type Diet is balanced: each one includes foods from the three basic food groups—protein, carbohydrates and fat—and all essential vitamins and minerals in the proportions necessary for good health. None of them is an extreme or fad diet which emphasizes one food group at the expense of others.

But even beyond the balance you would demand for health, the Body Type Diet takes into account the variation of nutritional requirements among body types. Thyroid and pituitary types, for example, need to get a larger proportion of their calories from protein than from carbohydrates, while adrenal and gonadal types need to draw more of their calories from carbohydrates. Pituitary types draw little or no calories from dairy products, while gonadal types can obtain a high proportion of their protein requirement from this source. Thyroid and adrenal types fall between the two extremes.

Taking these variations into account, the Body Type Diet differs as to the *source* of various nutrients. The diet for adrenal types, for example, takes more of its protein from whole grains and dairy products, and the diet for pituitary types from animal products. But none neglects any element that is essential to a healthy way of eating.

THE RATE OF
WEIGHT LOSS

Weight loss on this diet sequence occurs at the maximum safe rate for each individual. You can determine the weight *you* will lose by a simple formula. You will lose up to four percent of your body weight in the first week and up to two percent of your body weight in each of the following weeks. For example, suppose you weigh 150 pounds. You will lose up to six pounds the first week (four percent of 150), and up to three pounds in each week following (two percent of 150).

RULE #3: TIME YOUR EATING ACCORDING TO YOUR BODY TYPE.

When you eat is nearly as important, in dieting, as *what* you eat. Each of the body types has a rhythm, a time of day when the dominant gland is most active and a time of day when it is least active. It is easy for a dieter *not* to eat during the time of maximum activity of the dominant gland; conversely, it is hard to avoid snacking during the time of least activity. The actual burning of fat takes place more efficiently during the gland's active times.

Understanding the metabolic rhythms of each body type resolves an old dieting controversy about breakfast. Some dieting experts say that breakfast is a must, others that it's a "must not." The truth is that for some body types, a good breakfast is essential to efficient dieting; for others, it's the surest way to sabotage a diet. Pituitary and thyroid types diet more easily and lose weight more quickly if they eat a substantial breakfast with protein. Adrenal and gonadal types, on the other hand, do best if they eat more lightly in the morning and more substantially later in the day.

RULE #4: USE YOUR BODY TYPE HERBAL HELPS.

There are many doctors who believe that medicine began with the discovery of modern drugs, and overlook the older, less well-studied medicaments, such as herbs. I believe, however, that traditional herbal remedies have a great deal to offer, even to modern medicine. I've tested the use of herbs with my diet patients, and have found that there is an herbal tea for each body type which provides invaluable help in promoting dieting effectiveness.

Precisely how these herbs produce their effects is not entirely clear. Traditionally, Fenugreek Tea, which I use for pituitary types, is an intestinal lubricant and is used to relieve fevers, headaches, and irritation of the mucous membranes. Raspberry Leaf Tea (my tea for thyroid types) is used as an antacid. Parsley Tea (the adrenal type herbal help) is used for diseases of the kidney and for jaundice, and Red Clover Tea, which I use for gonadal types, is a blood purifier and diuretic which is also said to stimulate the liver and gall bladder.

Whatever their precise interaction with the glandular system, what the teas do for their respective body types is to produce a general systemic soothing effect which can probably be attributed to a soothing of the dominant gland. I have patients drink a cup of their herbal tea at the point in their day when their dominant gland is most likely to be irritated or fatigued—again, the time of day when the temptation to "snack" is greatest. The result: dieting is easier, cravings are less bothersome, hunger is easier to deal with, and "dieting nerves" are soothed and comforted.

RULE #5: USE THE BODY TYPE SNACKING STRATEGY.

Sometimes, even while you're dieting, you *will* feel a craving and you *will* take a snack. This is not supposed to happen—but it does. Most diets ignore this fact of life, but the Body Type Diet takes a more constructive approach: it deals with the biochemical reality underlying the so-called sin.

The desire to snack is not a random occurrence; it is related to the rhythm of the dominant gland. Each of the four major glands has a time of day when it is at its lowest ebb, and this produces a "danger" time of day when energy is low and the desire for an energy "lift" the hardest to resist. It is all too easy, at this time, to reach for one of the foods containing a stimulant for your dominant gland. But if, instead, you know of a food to eat that will support another of your glands in a gentle, healthy way, you will get the energy lift your body is crying for, with a minimum of harm to your diet.

The Body Type Snacking Strategy provides you with a snacking food for those danger times, one which is in harmony with your metabolic needs and which you can eat safely without destroying your diet. The actual snack that works differs according to body type, but the Body Type Snacking Strategy is used (with great success) by all the body types.

3

IRRESISTIBLE CRAVINGS

WHAT THEY TELL YOU ABOUT YOUR BODY TYPE

"What are the foods that you find yourself craving when you are on a diet?" I asked a woman patient who was about twenty pounds overweight. Her extra pounds were distributed all over her body, like baby fat.

"Oh, just the usual things," she said. "Yogurt, apples, cheese."

Intrigued by this reply (since I don't think I've ever craved any of these foods in my life), I asked the next patient which foods she had cravings for when dieting. This patient happened to be a woman with a slim face and slender legs, arms and hands, who was carrying her fifteen extra pounds around her hips and thighs. "Cookies and cake, especially with coffee," she said promptly, looking surprised that I should bother to ask. "Doesn't everyone?"

The next overweight patient that day happened to be a stocky, thickly built man with a paunch and a good deal of extra weight across his back as well. I asked him which he craved more strongly, yogurt or cookies. He looked at me as if I must be suffering from a touch of the sun. "I'm not a dessert person," he said, "and I don't even know what yogurt tastes like. I crave meat. Give me a good thick steak, and you can keep the rest of it."

I was fascinated by the diversity of these replies, and thought I'd heard everything, but there was more to come. Right after the stocky meat-lover came a woman who, from a sitting position, didn't look overweight at all. When she stood, however, I could see that she had all of ten extra pounds on her rear end. "I crave anything fried," she replied promptly to my question, "or creamy or spicy. The richer and hotter a food is, the less able I am to resist it."

Since that day I have asked this question of literally thousands of patients, and a pattern of cravings has long ago become clear. Cravings differ greatly from person to person, and it takes an understanding of body types to find a pattern in this diversity.

In fact, the diversity of cravings is one of the most important clues to the necessity of designing different diets for different body types, for in each body type the particular craving tells us exactly what is going on in the metabolism.

Cravings are irresistible desires for food, usually fattening food, which are the leading cause of dieting failure. The onset of a craving in the course of a diet is a definite sign that you are not following the right diet for your body type.

A craving is the body's way of saying that it needs something your diet is not supplying. Unfortunately, a craving is not specific. It's more like a baby's cry—a way of communicating a need, but not of saying what the need is. The body doesn't have a way of saying, "I need more protein!" or "Give me more Vitamin C!" or "I can't take all this coffee!" All it can do is say, "I need something!"

Almost invariably, we interpret the craving incorrectly. We feed ourselves potato chips when we need milk, or ice cream when we need eggs. The underlying need remains unsatisfied, and the craving continues though we stuff ourselves with food.

Neither a psychological nor a behavioral approach to cravings is truly effective. You can follow all the rules, eat slowly, chew everything a hundred times, eat only in the dining room with the television off, you can find more love and approval and go through years of therapy—and all this may improve your life a great deal. But if your *nutritional* requirements aren't satisfied by your diet, you will still have the physical needs that send you to the refrigerator. The only way to truly eliminate cravings is to get on a diet that meets your needs—that is, your Body Type Diet.

This doesn't mean that on your Body Type Diet you will never feel the slightest desire for something you shouldn't eat.

Desires can always arise. But there is a difference between a desire and a craving. A desire can be resisted, or it can be satisfied with a bite or two of what you want. A craving, because it is a sign of deficiency, can by its nature never be satisfied until the actual nutritional deficiency is satisfied.

FOOD GROUPS AND THE DOMINANT GLAND

Many patients have told me that when they've had cravings, they've felt instinctively that their bodies must be signaling that they have some requirement or other. But the object of the craving is never identical with the body's requirement; rather, the object of a craving has to do with the type of metabolism one has—that is, one's body type.

The explanation of why the four body types have cravings for different classes of foods lies in the biochemistry of how foods interact with the different glands. A number of discoveries, some recent and some of long standing, indicate that different foods actually stimulate different glands to become more active and to produce more of their particular chemicals, or hormones. In each of the four types, foods are craved which have a stimulating effect on the dominant gland.

In the pituitary type, cravings are invariably for dairy products, which recent research indicates are stimulating to the pituitary gland. In the thyroid type, cravings are for sweets and starches, which have long been known to stimulate the thyroid gland. The adrenal type craves animal products and salty foods, which stimulate the adrenal glands, and the gonadal type craves fats and spices, which are stimulating to the sex glands.

THE NATURAL AFFINITY FOR STIMULATING FOODS

In each body type, a natural affinity exists for the food group which stimulates the dominant gland. Because we each derive energy most easily from the gland which is strongest in our metabolism, the food which stimulates that gland naturally gives us the most effective energy "lift." We learn very early that foods which stimulate our dominant gland are the foods which will revive us most effectively whenever we feel tired, stressed, or run down.

We are all subject to many stresses—physical, mental, psychological, or any combination of these. If we have any nutritional deficiencies in the diet, this in itself is stressful. In addition, modern life imposes stresses of all kinds every day. One of the ways most of us react to stress is by *overeating* those foods which appear to relieve our stress and increase our energy—that is, those foods which stimulate our dominant gland.

This is the way in which cravings develop from our natural affinity for certain foods. What we are actually craving is not the nutritional value of what we crave, but its value as a *stimulant* to the dominant gland. This stimulating quality may not be bad in itself—what *is* bad is the way we come to overuse the stimulation, and thus to overeat.

Which comes first, the affinity for certain foods, or the body type? Does an infant who is fed thyroid-stimulating foods become a thyroid type, or does he or she have an inborn dominant thyroid gland which would become dominant no matter what he might be fed? The answer is that the body type is inborn, and is probably genetically determined. All infants begin their lives with the same diet—milk—yet evidence of body type can be seen very early, before differing diets would have had a chance to "force" an individual into one or the other of the body types.

DAIRY FOODS: THE PITUITARY STIMULATORS

Research on the pituitary gland has recently uncovered an intimate association between dairy products and pituitary gland activity. It appears that in infants, the pituitary hormone known as prolactin, a milk-stimulating hormone in the mother, is present in high concentrations in the baby's body and in the mother's milk which the baby drinks. The indications are that one function of milk is to stimulate pituitary activity in the baby and so promote brain development, since the hormone prolactin is critical in brain development and intellectual functioning.

If an infant is bottle-fed, he still receives significant amounts of prolactin from cow's milk. Studies have also shown that prolactin appears in higher-than-usual concentrations in the blood of adults who drink milk as well. Milk and milk products are thus clearly pituitary-gland stimulators, and people with dominant pituitary glands develop an affinity for milk and milk products very early. When under stress of any kind, they reach for milk products for their energy "lift," and thus come to actually crave these foods and to overeat them.

STARCHES: STIMULATING THE THYROID

The connection of stimulation of the thyroid with starch intake has long been established. Starches trigger a complicated series of events with two main results. One is that the thyroid is stimulated to produce more thyroid hormone, and the other is that the cells of the body, due to the presence of fructose in the blood, become less responsive to the presence of the thyroid hormone. The brain overreacts to the fructose and secretes still more thyroid-stimulating hormone (TSH). The thyroid gland is actually given a double dose of stimulation when starches are eaten—one from the initial direct stimulation, the second, some hours later, from TSH.

For a thyroid type, there seems to be no more effective energy lift than the one provided by a sweet or starch. Yet the danger of depending on these foods for stimulation, and so overeating, is very real.

MEAT, BUTTER, EGGS AND SALT: THE ADRENAL STIMULATORS

In the case of the adrenal glands, the biochemistry of food interaction has been the subject of intensive study lately due to the association of cholesterol (found in adrenal hormones) with heart disease. Cholesterol—the same cholesterol which is found in butter, meat, and eggs—is the core molecule of several adrenal hormones, such as cortisone and aldosterone. Eating cholesterol-rich foods stimulates the adrenal glands to produce its hormones in greater quantities.

Adrenal types derive stimulation from their adrenal hormones in several ways. For one, cortisone gives a feeling of energy and euphoria. It also helps adrenal types burn up tremendous food energy, one reason why A-types have such excellent digestions. Adrenal hormones also raise blood pressure, and there is a peculiar feeling of fullness and power associated with a rise in blood pressure, a feeling which adrenal types come to enjoy without really knowing what it is. Unfortunately, high blood pressure is associated with heart disease, to which adrenal types are particularly prone.

Salt also contributes to high blood pressure, and for this reason adrenal types often use it as a stimulant—again, with results that can be very damaging.

SPICES, FATS AND OILS: THE GONADAL STIMULATORS

It has long been known that spices have an effect called vasodilation which affects the gonads, or sex glands, in particular. Vasodilation is, simply, the effect of dilating the blood vessels and producing a state of passive congestion. When a G-type woman eats spicy foods the blood flow to the pelvic organs—uterus, vagina, ovaries as well as lower bowel—increases, resulting in stimulation of the function in these areas. These are two results: The area becomes more active and sensitive, and the production of hormones is increased. Eating fats also has an engorging effect on the pelvic organs; again, the result is stimulation of the sex glands.

Gonadal type women are not necessarily "oversexed." Sexual stimulation is a complex phenomenon and depends on many physical and psychological factors, not simply on the sex glands per se. On the contrary, G-type women tend to reach for spicy or creamy *foods* as a way of reviving their energy—with the result that overweight is common in this body type.

STRESS, OVERSTIMULATION, AND CRAVINGS: YOUR "DOWNFALL FOODS"

For each of the four body types, then, there is a particular class of foods which is stimulating to the dominant gland—one which forces it to produce more than usual of its particular hormones, and which gives to that body type a feeling of stimulation and energy resulting from the increased activity of the gland.

As with any stimulant, the foods which stimulate the dominant gland are needed in ever-greater quantities. At first, for example, a thyroid type may get an effective lift from one candy bar. Later it takes two or three, or a dozen, to produce the same effect. An adrenal type will need increasing quantities of rich, salty meats, a gonadal type more and more spicy foods, a pituitary type greater and greater amounts of cheese and ice cream.

What is happening within the body is a gradual weakening of the dominant gland. As the dominant gland becomes weaker, we eat more and more of our stimulating foods. The result is an ever-increasing cycle of overeating and its concomitant, overweight.

If you are overweight, you are unquestionably suffering from a weakened condition of the dominant gland. This condition can be corrected by either eliminating or drastically reducing foods which are stimulating to the dominant gland. Foods that stimulate your dominant gland are the "downfall foods" for your body type, for they are the ones with the greatest power to undermine and sabotage your dieting efforts.

Of course, dairy products, starches, meats and fats all have nutritional value, and all may be part of the diet in a healthy, non-overweight person. But you, being overweight, crave and consume your "danger foods" in quantities much beyond what you actually require. *You are using these foods as drugs, not as foods.* This is why you must restrict them in your diet until you have reestablished metabolic balance and eliminated the cravings, and use them only very circumspectly after you have reached your ideal weight.

On the other hand, it is not necessary for you to be as

concerned about foods which are not danger foods for your body type. In "for-everyone" diets, adrenal types may be told to eliminate starches, or thyroid types to cut out red meat, creating needless difficulty for the dieter. These foods are not addictive to these body types and it is possible to eat them without harm to the diet.

However, careful control of danger foods *is* necessary, and it is very difficult unless you first succeed in eliminating your cravings for them. Overcoming cravings is the essential key to becoming and remaining slender and healthy. You can only do this on a diet which satisfies your body's nutritional needs, as opposed to its needs for stimulation. Your Body Type Diet will strengthen your entire system, using foods which are nonstimulating to your dominant gland. It will also help you handle the normal stresses of living by strengthening your body's less-active glands, so that you do not need to rely on your dominant gland so exclusively for energy.

In the next chapter I will go through the four body types one by one, and show you in more detail the way its cravings come about and can be eliminated. I want you to understand this perfectly *before* you start to focus completely on your own body type.

4

BODY TYPE DIETING

HOW IT USES YOUR STRENGTHS AND CORRECTS YOUR WEAKNESSES

Before we go about finding your body type, let me give you some case histories from my medical files, illustrating how patients of each body type have responded to the diet which is right for their body type and their body type alone. These studies illustrate how the Body Type Diet works, by making use of the biochemical realities of the metabolism. In every case the diet has been designed to support the strengths and correct the weaknesses that are found in each of the four types of metabolism.

THE GONADAL TYPE: "WHY DOES IT ALWAYS GO *THERE?*"

Gretchen M. came to me about forty pounds overweight. I had known her for years and was surprised to see her in that state, for I had been to her wedding five years before and remembered a well-shaped gonadal type. She'd been a little too round in the rear, perhaps, but was by no means fat.

Now her rear had grown all out of proportion, as had her thighs. She had a good deal of cellulite—wrinkly fat which is particularly hard to lose—in these areas as well. She was very unhappy about the way she looked.

21

When I told her she had a problem typical of the gonadal-type woman, she looked embarrassed by the term, so I explained to her that being a "gonadal type" did not mean that she was in any sense overly sexual, or anything like that. It simply meant that the style of her body chemistry was set by the abundance of female sex hormones her system produced, and that this made her fat tend to accumulate in what is usually known as a very feminine location—the rear end.

The truth is that nature has not intended the G-type woman to have a flat rear. The gonads (or sex glands, which in woman are the ovaries), are the strongest gland in this body type, which means that they have a strong supply of female sex hormones in their systems. Sex hormones are the chemicals responsible for the development of sexual differences between men and women: under their direction woman acquire thicker hair, softer skin, finer features, rounder bodies, shorter stature, higher voices and more developed breasts. They also develop a more pronounced rear end—and in G-types this is the primary location of any extra pounds. However, it is *not* necessary for G-type women to be fat or out of proportion, as Gretchen now was.

She told me she had three children. The first two were born two years apart and the youngest had come along only fifteen months after the second child. I suspected immediately that she had exhausted her sex glands through the stress of such closely spaced childbearing.

When I asked about her cravings, she told me what she couldn't resist was ice cream. She thought it was a healthy dessert and often gave it to her children, so it was always in the house. With three children under five she was very overtired, and she'd have a dish of it to keep going. She only ate the creamiest, high butterfat kind. Another downfall was Mexican food. "My husband loves it," she explained lamely, "so of course when he wants to go out I have to keep him company."

Obviously, Gretchen was using gonadal-stimulating foods—spicy and creamy food—as a means of keeping herself going. I recommended that she try to get a bit more rest, and put her on the Gonadal Type Diet. It is a diet high in complex carbohydrates and low in animal protein, carefully designed to avoid further stimulation to the sex glands.

Two weeks later she had lost eleven pounds. When she asked me whether reducing stimulation to her sex glands through diet would reduce her sexual responsiveness, I replied that sexual response is a complex phenomenon which is not tied solely to sex hormones. However, the fatigue she had been feeling, and which her Body Type Diet would correct, was certainly not conducive to a happy sex life.

She went on to lose her forty pounds in about fourteen weeks. To her delight her rear is now once more nicely rounded and youthful, although it is not and will never be boyish and flat. When I asked about her husband's reaction to her new shape, she smiled and said that what he really appreciated was her improved energy level! She didn't wink but I got the message.

I told her that I wanted her to continue on the G-Type Health and Weight Maintenance Diet indefinitely. This diet does allow for some spicy food in moderation, but she would always be wise to avoid overeating from these gonad-stimulating foods. By doing so she would be taking timely steps towards keeping off the cellulite which, in her body type, is always apt to accumulate on the rear and upper thighs.

THE MODEL'S PROBLEM

Occasionally I see a gonadal type who has only a small amount of fat to lose. Barbara was and is a top model; you have seen her picture many times in magazines, wearing bikinis and other revealing bits of clothing. Many clothing manufacturers like the look of a slightly accentuated rear end, for it shows certain clothes to advantage.

But Barbara had a real problem, considering her profession: her thighs and her rear end had begun to spread and to show cellulite. Although women of all body types, and a few men, are susceptible to cellulite, gonadal type women are the most susceptible to it of all. Barbara admitted that she had been on an extended spree of rich and creamy food. Now, for the first time, she was having trouble getting work. The camera never lies, and in her line of work cellulite is a bitter truth.

I saw my treatment of her as an acid test of the Gonadal Type Diet. The cellulite removal had to be absolutely complete. Other people can get away with a trace of wrinkly fat; she couldn't. Since she had only twelve pounds to lose, she went on the Weight Loss Diet for two weeks and then the G-Type Last Five Pounds Diet for a week. I had her lose fifteen pounds, just to make sure all the cellulite was gone. It did disappear. The benefits of the G-Type Diet are not just for people like Barbara, of course, but her case illustrates the way the diet works for someone with the motivation to follow it religiously.

THE ADRENAL TYPE: IS FAT INEVITABLE?

There are certain phrases, meant to be comforting, that actually hurt more than they comfort. Phrases like, "Don't worry about your weight—you carry it so well." "You're not fat, you're muscular." "You're athletic-looking." "You're built like your father" (especially depressing if you happen to be a woman). And, perhaps worst of all, "You're just big-boned."

The object of these remarks is invariably an adrenal type, the person whose strongest gland is the powerful adrenal gland. Or, I should say, adrenal glands, for there are two of them, one located on top of each kidney. Though no bigger than two lima beans, the adrenals are the most powerful gland of the body and the ones with the most diverse functions.

Chemicals secreted by the adrenals, which go by the general name of adrenal hormones, assist the liver in the manufacture of glycogen, the blood sugar which is later distributed throughout the body by the thyroid. They assist the kidneys to purify the body's fluids. They control the formation of both muscle and fat, and affect the balance between them. They also stimulate the appetite, so that we eat and keep our bodies supplied with food. The adrenals are the glands of balance, power and steadiness of energy, and contribute these qualities to many functions of the metabolism.

The adrenal-type metabolism shares the characteristics of its dominant gland. A-types are the most powerful and steadiest of the four body types. Adrenal types even look powerful: they are solidly built, have square or round faces, strong, squarish hands and feet, broad shoulders, and thick waists—bodies shaped for power rather than speed.

In their cravings A-types are the amazement of other body types in that they truly do not care about dessert. The adrenals are stimulated by salty foods, especially salty meats, which have the effect of increasing the production of adrenal hormones. One of their effects is to raise the blood pressure, which produces a feeling of pressure and energy in the body, and this is the feeling to which A-types are unconsciously addicted. The quick energy "rush" of carbohydrates does little for them, and this is why desserts do not appeal. When A-types want energy it is red meat that turns them on.

The adrenals are powerful glands, and A-types do not tire easily. Yet they like to keep that powerful feeling going, and it is not unusual for an A-type to eat three hearty, meat-laden meals per day, with salty snacks (peanuts, salami, aged cheese) in between.

The combination of the powerful, strongly built body, the strong fame that carries weight well, the strong digestion which adrenal types always enjoy, and the healthy appetite that adrenal hormones produce, makes overweight almost inevitable in A-types. But it is a mistake to imagine that an A-type must be fat. There is great potential for a slender, well-balanced and much healthier body, but it requires a drastic change in eating habits.

The overweight A-type may acquire a figure of truly Falstaffian proportions. Take Robert S. I heard his booming voice in the waiting room before I saw him, and he had all the other patients laughing. He is a good-looking man, with great energy, verve and an infectiously charming personality—and eighty extra pounds. I knew at once he was an adrenal type, for this body type has its own typical fat distribution. Where thyroid types balloon around the middle and remain slim in their arms and legs, A-types thicken all over, though they do put a great deal of their excess weight in front, in a pot belly.

Robert was a high-powered salesman who put in long hours and often had to share meals with customers as part of making a sale. I saw from his high energy level that although he was in the habit of overstimulating his adrenals, he had not exhausted them. (The adrenals, fortunately, are much harder to exhaust than the thyroid or the pituitary, and can stand a great deal of overstimulation). When adrenal types decide to diet, their strong adrenals will help them lose weight faster than any other body type.

Not surprisingly, dieting came fairly easily to Robert, despite the fact that he had never before tried to curb his appetite. Even as a child, he told me, his mother had never discouraged him from eating, since he was eating "healthy" meat and potatoes rather than "unhealthy" sweets. Thanks to his strong adrenals, his energy remained high on the A-Type Weight Loss Diet despite the reduction in adrenal stimulators. The first week Robert weighed in to find he had lost seventeen pounds! He proceeded to lose the rest of his eighty extra pounds in only twelve weeks, and he kept laughing the whole time. I have rarely had such a delightful patient. On the twelfth week of his diet he brought in with him the trousers he had been wearing the first day. He had put them on over his new clothes, and they were yards too big.

INCREASED CREATIVITY: THE A-TYPE DIET BONUS

In about the third week of his diet Robert reported that he seemed to be becoming more creative and spontaneous in his work. I explained that this was due to the increased pituitary and thyroidal activity in his metabolism. These glands give lightness and quickness to the system, and these qualities are reflected in a more creative mental and emotional state.

Robert's last five pounds came off as easily as the others, on the A-Type Last Five Pounds Diet. He is now on the A-Type Health and Weight Maintenance Diet, and tells me that he feels great and is an even more successful salesman than before. His cheerful gusto is now balanced with greater creativity and flexibility—an unbeatable combination.

We tend to associate the "meat, no dessert" craving only with men, but there are many adrenal-type women in this world as well. The A-type woman also gains weight across the middle and is prone to acquire a pot belly and to lose her waist when overweight. She is also what Jane Russell refers to as a "full-figured gal," and puts on weight very readily in her breasts.

Sonya J., a teenager, was already thirty pounds overweight at the age of sixteen. With her stocky, full-figured body she looked a good deal older than her years. I could see that her adrenals were going full blast and that this was allowing very little activity to her thyroid or pituitary. So I took the drastic step of putting her on a completely vegetarian diet, with instructions to her mother to be sure that she got plenty of protein from dairy products and eggs.

I did not see her again for several months, and when I did I barely knew her. The transformation was both stunning and delightful. She was slim and her body had much more lightness and grace. Her face now showed a fine bone structure which had previously been lost in a jowly accumulation of fat.

A vegetarian diet is by no means ideal for everyone. But for adrenal types, particularly adrenal-type women, the nearly vegetarian diet is ideal. Lacking a pronounced sweet tooth, they are not tempted to eat too many sweets, and their strong adrenals do not suffer in the least from the lack of stimulation. At the same time the stimulation this diet gives to the pituitary and thyroid provides an excellent degree of balance to their metabolism. In Sonya's case and in many other A-type patients, the results have been very gratifying.

THE THYROID TYPE: WHEN A THIN PERSON GETS FAT

The overweight thyroid type is among the commonest sights in a doctor's life. The thyroid type is intended by nature to be slim—every line of the body calls out to be lithe, shapely and delicate. Yet this is a metabolic type highly vulnerable to overweight, with a dominant gland easily exhausted and particularly susceptible to the inducements of our sweets-oriented eating habits.

The thyroid, located at the base of the throat just above the notch you can feel in the front of the breastbone, is in charge of the function of the metabolism called *oxidation*—the burning of food in the tissues. Like all the glands, it works by secreting chemicals called hormones into the bloodstream. The amount of thyroid hormone this gland secretes determines the rate at which the body burns its food. Thyroid hormones also control the flow of energy from the liver to the blood. The liver is our storehouse of glycogen, or blood sugar, and it releases this energy supply into the blood when directed to do so by the thyroid. In addition the thyroid affects heart rate and muscle tone.

With the thyroid as dominant gland, the thyroid type has, ideally, an abundant supply of thyroid hormones, which in turn produce a metabolism which burns food rapidly and efficiently. It also produces a body which has a streamlined, "greyhound" look—slender arms and legs, long, slim hands and feet, a long neck, a neat, slim torso. Even in an overweight T-type, traces of this basically slender body type always remain. They get fat around the middle, but fat seldom goes below their thighs—the calves and feet always look as if they belonged to another, slimmer person, and their hands and face remain thin until they become very overweight indeed. An overweight T-type never looks like a "fat person," but rather like a slim person who has, unaccountably, become fat!

Slender T-types are the ones who are the envy of their friends for their ability to eat and eat and not gain weight, an ability that lasts only as long as the thyroid remains strong. They are wiry, speedy and energetic, and they never need to rest—or so they think. Unfortunately, they generally overrate their staying power. The truth is that T-types do need to rest, because of the nature of the thyroid itself. The gland is designed to provide the body with "bursts" of energy, but it needs time to recover after a release of thyroid hormones. T-types do have great energy bursts, but they should intersperse these bursts with periods of rest.

Instead, what they tend to do—and I have seen this over and over in both my medical and my weight-control patients—is to take a quick-acting thyroid stimulant like sugar, coffee, cola or tea whenever they begin to feel tired. Of course, all body types tend to take foods which stimulate our dominant gland whenever we feel tired, pressured or stressed, but T-types are unusually vulnerable to this tendency.

The result is predictable. The thyroid, constantly stimulated, begins to become less efficient. In extreme cases it may even collapse and stop functioning altogether. The T-type, used to eating whatever she or he wants and not gaining weight, now finds that the pounds start to collect—and the transformation from slim to fat can be dramatically sudden.

THE SUDDEN ONSET OF
T-TYPE FAT

Sally H. is a typical thyroid type. I'd seen her about a year before, when she'd needed a minor surgical procedure. At that time she'd been very slender—in fact she was working as a model (many fashion models are T-types.) But this time when she walked into my office I nearly didn't recognize her. She weighed almost two hundred pounds. Her former striking looks were almost totally buried in the fat—although even at this point she still had trim ankles and feet. She looked extremely unhealthy and her whole body was covered with cellulite.

I learned that she had gone through a divorce a few months after her surgery. These two events, coming so close together, had added up to a great deal of stress, but instead of taking things easy for a time she'd reacted in typical T-type style and taken on a heavy work schedule. Then, feeling tired, she'd started drinking quantities of cola and eating thyroid-stimulating sweets. She even had to have a cola drink and a sweet before she could get up in the morning! In this way she had gained over ninety pounds, and her modeling work had of course evaporated.

I put her immediately on the Thyroid Type Diet—a high-protein diet with a minimum of starches and no caffeine whatever. I wanted to rest her highly overstimulated thyroid, and I also wanted to give some stimulation to her adrenals. For T-types who have been relying on thyroidal energy to get through their days, stimulating the adrenals is an important part of dieting because it brings these powerful glands, with their steadier energy, into action, and so takes a great deal of the burden off the thyroid.

Sally had trouble following her diet at first because of the severity of her thyroidal exhaustion. In her run-down state she imagined she couldn't function without stimulants, but after about a week she began to feel the strengthening of her adrenals. She continued dieting and lost weight at the steady rate of four pounds per week, until she had lost fifty pounds. At this point she suddenly began looking radiant again, and I knew that her thyroid was starting to recover. From this point on her weight loss became more rapid, the result of her more efficient thyroid. She lost her last pounds of excess weight on the T-Type Last Five Pounds Diet, and by the end of her diet she looked and felt completely herself again.

I warned her, however, that she would have to continue to be careful with her diet for the rest of her life. Although she was now much stronger she would always have the basically delicate thyroid-type metabolism. It responds beautifully to a healthy, high-protein, low-carbohydrate diet, but disastrously to overstimulation through sweets and caffeine.

THE T-TYPE ENERGY CONNECTION

Jerry S., a young and ambitious professional man who worked long hours, was another interesting thyroid type. When he came to me for help he was only about fifteen pounds overweight every pound of which was in a "roll" around his midsection. But his real problem was the unsteadiness of his energy. I asked for his dietary history, and it was a thyroidal nightmare. Breakfast was coffee and toast. Next came a coffee break, with doughnut, at midmorning. Lunch was a sandwich, a coke, another coffee and a dessert, and he told me that often by the end of the day he was too tired to make dinner, and just had coffee and cookies.

When I told him I was taking him off caffeine and sweets, his eyes flashed angrily (this was his addiction to thyroid stimulants making itself known). He'd imagined I was going to prescribe diet pills, which T-types love because they are also thyroid stimulants and give them a temporary feeling that they have their old energy back. I told him diet pills were the last thing he needed in his condition—I doubted his thyroid could take much more strain.

He was an intelligent man, and when I explained to him what he was doing to his metabolism he agreed to try and change his eating habits. I had him reduce his caffeine intake gradually over the course of a week, until he was down to just one cup of decaffeinated coffee which I allowed him in the morning.

He lost his fifteen pounds in three weeks. The roll of fat

around his middle gave way to firm flesh, and his complexion, which had been dull-looking, became smoother and more luminous. He reported that he was no longer getting tired in the middle of the day. He needed less sleep, and was able to put in the long hours his work required without a break.

THE TEMPTATIONS OF
THE T-TYPE

I emphasized to both Sally and Jerry, and to all my T-type patients, the importance of continuing attention to diet and to rest. Given the constant availability of sweets and starches, and the social lures of a cup of coffee, tea or cola, this warning is necessary. T-types who have lost their excess weight and balanced their metabolisms can enjoy caffeine in moderation, can even eat some sweets, but should always be attentive not to rely on these stimulants for energy when what their bodies really need is a period of rest.

THE PITUITARY
TYPE: "I'M TOO OLD
TO HAVE BABY
FAT!"

Sarah K. said she was thirty-seven, but from her looks she could have been in her late twenties. I noticed first that her head gave the appearance of being slightly too big for her body, a sure sign of a pituitary type. She also had a round, childlike face and a bright, interested expression. Her thirty or so extra pounds were in the typical "baby-fat" all-over distribution of the P-type—that is, she had some fat on her hands and arms, her back and chest were rather pudgy and her stomach was rounded like a child's. She did not have one particular area of fat, such as hips, thighs or rear; all were rounded but no one area stood out noticeably. All in all, a classic P-type—and an overweight one.

Sarah told me that she was a vegetarian. The reason, she said, was that her digestion was weak, especially for heavy foods like meat, so she generally avoided animal foods and obtained most of her protein from dairy products. "In fact," she said, "I almost live on yogurt and cheese sandwiches. I didn't think it would be possible to get fat on yogurt, but it looks like I've done it!"

When I gave her the Pituitary Type Diet, she looked non-plussed. The diet contains the highest proportion of protein of any of the diets. It also allows no dairy products at all, and has meat at every meal including breakfast.

Sarah was reluctant to try the diet at first, but I was able to persuade her that while a vegetarian diet is suitable for some body types, it is not appropriate for the P-type metabolism. She promised to try it for a week.

When I saw her the following week she was beaming over a weight loss of five pounds. At this point she was ready to hear an explanation of how and why the diet works. I told her that being a pituitary type means that of her body's four major glands, the pituitary was the strongest and was the one which set the tone of her metabolism. It is located within the skull behind the eyes, and is known as the "master gland" because it is responsible for controlling and regulating all glandular activity.

The pituitary works by secreting chemicals, called pituitary hormones, into the bloodstream. These hormones regulate the activity of the thyroid and the adrenals, and have general control over the functioning of the sex glands as well. They are responsible for the body's growth and sexual maturation. They also govern the body's response to changes in the external environment. Through a complex series of chemical reactions, the pituitary reacts to such aspects of the environment as the weather and the time of day, and conveys these changes to the rest of the body so that it can respond to them in an appropriate way.

A metabolism which is dominated by this master gland has, by nature, very good coordination among the different parts of the body. But there is no one aspect of the body's metabolism that works more strongly than any other. This explains why fat, in the P-type, accumulates all over the body. Each of the other glands has a particular area where it directs fat to be stored. In the pituitary type, no one area is emphasized, so fat is stored every-where more or less equally. This produces the typical baby-fat look of the P-type.

Sarah had already told me that her digestion was somewhat

weak; I now learned that her sexual function also was not strong. She said she'd never been able to understand what all the "fuss about sex" was about. Both these weaknesses can be traced to the typical weakness of the P-type metabolism—a lack of strength in the adrenals (digestion) and the gonads (sexual function). She'd been overstimulating her pituitary, and giving a corresponding understimulation to her "lower" glands.

To offset these weaknesses, the Pituitary Type Diet employs a high proportion of animal protein, which is stimulating to the lower glands. Without this stimulation the metabolism remains sluggish in the essential adrenal and gonadal functions. And without strong support of the lower glands, pituitary types easily become fatigued and stressed and feel uncontrollable cravings for dairy foods. On the Pituitary Type Diet, these cravings are drastically reduced and, after a few weeks, entirely eliminated.

I saw Sarah every week for the next ten weeks. She lost an average of three pounds per week, until she reached her weight goal of 120 pounds. What impressed her was how easily she dieted; she was free of cravings and felt more energetic than before she started dieting. What impressed me, on the other hand, was observing her metabolism's balance improve as the weeks went by. She lost her baby fat and began to look more like an "adult." And as she slimmed down, she developed a more sensual shape. At the same time her digestion improved, and she told me with some surprise that she was starting to understand why people were so interested in sex! For Sarah, the Pituitary Type diet is the *only* diet that would produce the positive and holistic benefits that so delighted us both.

ANOTHER WAY P-TYPES
CAN GO WRONG

A P-type I saw about three years ago was an attorney who felt that he would be more effective in front of juries if he were slimmer. So he'd (unwisely) eaten nothing for the past two weeks but grapefruit and cottage cheese. He was now worried about his health, and well he might be—he had lost seven pounds but felt weak and was suffering from headaches and irritability.

Since he was a pituitary type, his problem was easily explained. The diet he'd been on couldn't have been worse for his body type. Pituitary types need plenty of animal protein and must avoid dairy products completely—the exact opposite of what he'd been doing.

I changed him at once to the P-Type Weight Loss Diet. Two weeks later he was back with a glowing report. He'd lost five more pounds and was now at his ideal weight. But of equal or greater importance was the fact that his weakness and headaches were gone. His very appearance proclaimed the increased metabolic balance produced by his Body Type Diet.

NOW IT'S YOUR TURN

Now, the time has come for you to start applying these principles to your own weight problem. In the next chapter I take you through the simple steps of finding your body type. Once you have done this, you will be ready to start the Weight Loss Program for your body type.

5

THE BODY
TYPE CHECK
LIST

FINDING YOUR
BODY TYPE

To select your Body Type Diet—the diet which will work for your own type of metabolism—you must first know what type of body yours is. Your "body type," as you have seen, is simply a short-hand way of describing your metabolism—its strengths and weaknesses, its needs and requirements—in terms of which of the four major glands dominates your body chemistry. This chapter will show you exactly how to discover whether your dominant gland is the gonads, the adrenal glands, the thyroid gland or the pituitary gland, by means of simple observations you can make of yourself, and *without* using costly and time-consuming laboratory tests.

What makes it possible to determine your body type by simple self-observation is the pervasive influence of the dominant gland on many aspects of your makeup. The most important influence of the dominant gland is in your appearance: your *body's shape,* your *fat distribution* and the *location of your wrinkly fat,* or cellulite. Sections 1, 2 and 3 of the Body Type Check List focus on these three aspects of appearance. Because of their importance, most questions in these sections are worth two points in determining your body type. The fourteen illustrations which accompany the Check List will help you answer the questions in the first three sections.

Other influences of the dominant gland are in the areas of *food preference; energy level; bodily responses* to various situations; and the broad outlines of your *personality.* Sections 4, 5, 6 and 7 of the Body Type Check List focus on these areas. Since the dominant gland has a more variable influence on these areas than on your appearance, most questions in these sections are worth only one point in determining your body type.

Section 1, 2 and 3—those concerned with appearance— should be completed while standing before a full-length mirror in your underwear or, preferably, nude. If possible you should enlist the aid of a friend or spouse in answering the questions, since another person can view you from angles that are difficult to see on yourself. However, be sure that the person you ask to help you is the kind who will be frank. He or she should not be shy about helping you decide whether your hips are round or flat, or whether you have more fat on your stomach, hips or thighs. Don't pick a friend who will say what she thinks you want to hear. You need to hear the truth, because that's the only way you will be able to find out what's going on inside your body.

Keep in mind, while completing these sections, that there is no one way your body "should" look. There is only the way that is characteristic of your body type. There is not one "perfect" type—the adrenal type is *different* from the thyroid, pituitary or gonadal type, not "better" or "worse." Each type has the potential to be perfect in its own unique way. The important thing is to know which type you *are!* Failure to recognize differences has been the cause of infinite confusion and lack of success in dieting in the past. Now is the time to end that confusion by finding your body type.

After completing the sections on appearance in front of the mirror, sit down and carefully complete the remaining sections. Again, be honest—there is nothing to gain and everything to lose by pretending to be someone you aren't. Finally, when you have finished the test, complete the Scoring Instructions and you will know your body type.

There are separate Check Lists for women and men. This is because of the fact that there are four body types in women and only three types in men. Also, cellulite location is a good indicator of body type in women but not in men; therefore Section 3, which focuses on cellulite, appears only in the Check List for Women. The Body Type Check List for Women begins below; the Check List for Men begins on page 54.

THE BODY TYPE
CHECK LIST FOR
WOMEN

SECTION 1: BODY SHAPE AND APPEARANCE

1. Look at yourself straight on in the mirror, focusing on the overall outline and shape of your body.

a. My body is at least a full size smaller above the waist than below. (See Figure 1, page 65)

Two points for G: ___

b. My body is stocky and full-figured, without a pronounced curve at waist or hips. (See Figure 3, page 67)

Two points for A: ___

c. My body is curvy but much fuller through the middle (waist, hips and upper thighs) than at the extremities (neck and head, lower arms, calves and ankles). (See Figure 5, page 69)

Two points for T: ___

d. My body is childlike in outline, with small breasts and "baby fat" all over. (See Figure 7, page 71)

Two points for P: ___

2. Now turn sideways to the mirror and focus on the line of your back.

a. My back is slightly "swayed" and my rear end sticks out prominently. (See Figure 2, page 66)

Two points for G: ___

b. My back is straight and my rear appears to be flat and "tucked under." (See Figure 4, page 68)

Two points for A: ___

c. My rear is round but not extremely pronounced; my lower back is straight. (See Figure 6, page 70)

Two points for T: ___

d. My rear is small and childlike, my shoulders are round and my head comes forward from the line of my back. (See Figure 8, page 72)

Two points for P: ___

3. Next, focus on your head—its shape
and its relation to your body size.

a. My head is slightly small for my   Two points for G: _✓_
body size.

b. My head is squarish and I have a   Two points for A: __
square or round face.

c. My head is long and I have a slender Two points for T: __
face.

d. My head is slightly large for my body Two points for P: __
size.

4. Examine your hands and feet. They
are:

a. Average in size, small fingers and   Two points for G: _✓_
toes.

b. Square, with small fingers and toes. Two points for A: __

c. Long, with tapering fingers and toes. Two points for T: __

d. Small, delicate.   Two points for P: __

5. Focus on your teeth. They are:

a. White, medium-sized, uneven.   Two points for G: _✓_

b. Large, slightly yellowish.   Two points for A: __

c. Small, white, even.   Two points for T: __

d. Large, especially front center.   Two points for P: __

6. Look at the shape of your mouth. It
is:

a. Thin, well-shaped.   Two points for G: ⎽✓⎽

b. Full.   Two points for A: ⎽⎽

c. Wide, mobile.   Two points for T: ⎽⎽

d. Rosebud.   Two points for P: ⎽⎽

7. Look at your skin. It is:
a. Smooth, oily.   Two points for G: ⎽⎽

b. Oily, slightly coarse.   Two points for A: ⎽⎽

c. Smooth, of normal oiliness.   Two points for T: ⎽✓⎽

d. dry, delicate.   Two points for P: ⎽⎽

8. Finally, think back to when you were
at your ideal weight, or try to imagine how you would look at your normal weight based on what you have
already observed about your present
shape. At your ideal weight you
would be:
a. Slim, but with curvy hips and rear.   Two points for G: ⎽✓⎽

b. Slender but full-figured and strongly Two points for A: ⎽⎽
built.
c. Very slender and fine-boned.   Two points for T: ⎽⎽

d. Slender, childlike and undeveloped.   Two points for P: ⎽⎽

Now add up your points for each type.
Total Score for Section 1:

G:⎽⎽⎽14⎽⎽⎽ A:⎽⎽⎽⎽⎽⎽ T:⎽⎽2⎽⎽⎽ P:⎽⎽⎽⎽⎽⎽

SECTION 2: FAT DISTRIBUTION

9. Look at yourself in the mirror, focusing on your excess weight. Where is
   most of your fat?
   a. On the rear end.   Two points for G: __

   b. Across the stomach and upper back.   Two points for A: __

   c. Around the middle—waist, hips, up-   Two points for T: ✓
      per thighs.
   d. All over, no single location.   Two points for P: __

10. Look at yourself from the back, or
    ask your friend to look. Do you have
    more fat:
    a. Below the waist.   Two points for G: ✓

    b. Across the upper back.   Two points for A: __

    c. Around the waist.   Two points for T: __

    d. All over—not more above or below.   Two points for P: __

11. Still looking at yourself from the
    back, do you have "saddlebags"
    (pockets of fat on the outer thighs)?
    a. Yes.   One point for G: __

       and   One point for T: __

    b. No.   One point for A: ✓

       and   One point for P: __

12. Turn back to look at yourself from the front again. Do you have a "spare tire" (a roll of fat around the middle)?

a. Yes.   One point for A: ✓

  and   One point for T: ___

b. No.   One point for G: ___

  and   One point for P: ___

13. Focus on your hands and feet. Do they have an accumulation of fat?

a. Yes.   One point for A: ___

  and   One point for P: ___

b. No.   One point for T: ✓

  and   One point for G: ___

Now add up your points for each type.
Total Score for Section 2:

G:____2____ A:____1____ T:____3____ P:_____

SECTION 3: CELLULITE DISTRIBUTION

To check for cellulite, first examine the area in question. Does the fat there appear to be wrinkly and "cottage cheesey"? If so, the area has cellulite. If the area appears to have fat but the fat is not wrinkly, then gently squeeze about an inch or so of the fat between two fingers, or have your friend do so. When you examine the fat in this way you may find wrinkles that were not apparent just from looking at it. If you do, the area does have cellulite, although it is cellulite at an earlier stage than cellulite you can see without squeezing it between your fingers, and you should count yourself as having cellulite in that location.

14. First, check your upper arms. Do
     you have cellulite?

a. Yes.   One point for A: ___

   and   One point for T: ___

b. No.   One point for G: ✓___

   and   One point for P: ___

15. Check your upper hips. Do you have
     cellulite?

a. Yes.   Two points for T: ___

b. No.   One point for G: ___

   and   One point for A: ／___

   and   One point for P: ___

16. Check your lower hips. Do you have cellulite?

a. Yes.   One point for G: ___

   and   One point for T: ___

b. No.   One point for A: ___

   and   One point for P: ___

17. Check your upper thighs. Do you have cellulite?

a. Yes.   Two points for T: ___

b. No.   One point for G: ___

   and   One point for A: ___

   and   One point for P: ___

18. Check your knees. Do you have cellulite?

a. Yes.   Two points for P: ___

b. No.   One point for G: ___

   and   One point for A: ___

   and   One point for T: ___

19. Check your upper back. Do you have cellulite?

a. Yes.   Two points for A: ___

b. No.   One point for G: ✓

   and   One point for T: ___

   and   One point for P: ___

20. Check your rear end. Do you have cellulite?

a. Yes   Two points for G: ✓

b. No.   One point for A: ___

   and   One point for T: ___

   and   One point for P: ___

21. What is your *main* area of cellulite?

a. Rear, outer thighs.   Two points for G: ✓

b. Stomach, back.   Two points for A: ___

c. Upper thighs.   Two points for T: ___

d. Knees, breasts.   Two points for P: ___

Now add up your points for each type.
Total Score for Section 3:

G:_____ A:_____ T:_____ P:_____

SECTION 4: FOOD PREFERENCES

22. Of the following foods, which do you
love the most?

a. Rich or spicy foods.   One point for G: ___

b. Steak, salty foods.   One point for A: ___

c. Bread, sweets.   One point for T: ___

d. Dairy products.   One point for P: ___ ✓

23. At a party, which of these foods
would you find hardest to resist?

a. The creamy dips.   One point for G: ___

b. The hot dogs, salami or peanuts.   One point for A: ___ ✓

c. The cakes or candies.   One point for T: ___

d. The ice cream or frozen yogurt.   One point for P: ___

24. How much coffee, tea or cola do you
drink each day?

a. One or two cups.   One point for G: ___

b. Three or four cups.   One point for A: ___ ✓

c. Five cups or more.   One point for T: ___

d. None or one cup.   One point for P: ___

25. Which of the following would you
prefer for breakfast?

a. French toast.   One point for G: ___

b. Bacon and eggs.   One point for A: ✓

c. Toast and jam.   One point for T: ___

d. Fruit and yogurt.   One point for P: ___

26. Ideally, when would you like to have
your biggest meal?

a. Breakfast.   One point for G: ___

b. Dinner.   One point for A: ✓

c. Lunch.   One point for T: ___

d. Prefer no big meal, just lots of snacks.   One point for P: ___

Now add up your points for each type.
Total Score for Section 4:

G:_____ A:___4_____ T:_____ P:___1_____

SECTION 5: ENERGY PATTERNS

27. Ideally, how many hours do you
sleep each night?

a. 8-9 hours.   One point for G: ___

b. 4-6 hours.   One point for A: ___

c. 5-6 hours when feeling good, 9-10   One point for T: ___
hours when tired.

d. 7-8 hours.   One point for P: _1_

28. When does your highest-energy period occur?

a. Late in the day. One point for G: ___

b. Energetic all day. One point for A: _/_

c. Following meals. One point for T: ___

d. First thing in the morning. One point for P: ___

29. Do you have trouble sleeping at night?

a. Rarely. One point for G: ___

b. Often. One point for A: ___

c. Occasionally, but only for one night at a time. One point for T: _/_

d. Occasionally, but when I do it happens every night for a while. One point for P: ___

Now add up your points for each type.
Total Score for Section 5:

G:_____ A:_____ T:____/____ P:_____

SECTION 6: BODILY RESPONSES

30. How much do you perspire?

a. Moderately, with exertion. One point for G: _/_

b. Quite a bit, even at rest. One point for A: ___

c. Variably. Very lightly when slim, more when heavy. One point for T: ___

d. Lightly. One point for P: ___

31. Are you prone to colds and allergies?

a. Not usually—only when tired.   One point for G: ___

b. No, almost never.   One point for A: _1_

c. Yes, quite a bit.   One point for T: ___

    and   One point for P: ___

32. Are you prone to upset stomach or diarrhea?

a. No.   One point for G: _1_

    and   One point for A: ___

b. Yes.   One point for T: ___

    and   One point for P: ___

33. Are you prone to headaches?

a. Rarely.   One point for G: _1_

    and   One point for A: ___

b. Occasionally.   One point for T: ___

c. Yes, quite a bit.   One point for P: ___

34. Do your hands and feet feel cold at night?

a. Sometimes, in cold weather.   One point for G: ___

    and   One point for P: ___

b. Rarely.   One point for A: _1_

c. Often.   One point for T: ___

35. When you are ill, which parts of your
   body are most likely to ache?

a. Hands and feet.   One point for G: ___

b. Lower back.   One point for A: _/_

c. Neck and shoulders.   One point for T: ___

d. Knees.   One point for P: ___

36. Which of your senses is the most
   important to you—that is, the one
   you use most in making up your mind
   about the qualities of an object?

a. Touch.   One point for G: ___

b. Hearing.   One point for A: ___

c. Taste/smell.   One point for T: ___

d. Sight.   One point for P: _/_

37. Which of your senses is the least important to you—that is, the one you
   weigh the least in judging an object?

a. Sight.   One point for G: ___

b. Taste/smell.   One point for A: ___

c. Hearing.   One point for T: ___

d. Touch.   One point for P: _/_

38. Are you prone to cramps during your menstrual period?

a. First day only.   One point for G: ___

b. Rarely.   One point for A: ___

c. Yes, quite badly.   One point for T: ___

d. Very little.   One point for P: _/_

39. If you have been pregnant, which of these best describes your experience?

a. Delightful—enjoyed it.   One point for G: ___

b. Easy, comfortable.   One point for A: ___

c. Felt heavy and uncomfortable.   One point for T: ___

d. Didn't like it much.   One point for P: ___

40. Ideally, how often would you like to make love?

a. Every day.   One point for G: _/_

b. Twice a week or so.   One point for A: ___

c. In spurts. A lot for a while, then not   One point for T: ___
at all for a while.

d. Once a week or less.   One point for P: ___

Now add up your points for each type.
Total Score for Section 6:

G:___ 2 ___ A:___ 3 ___ T:_____ P:___ 3 ___

SECTION 7: PERSONALITY TRAITS

41. Is it easy for you to laugh at yourself? (Be honest, now!)

a. Yes.   One point for G: ___

and   One point for T: ___

b. No.   One point for A: ___

and   One point for P: ___

42. Which of these subjects do you most enjoy discussing or thinking about?

a. Sex, home, family, food.   One point for G: ___

b. Business, money, practical things.   One point for A: ___

c. The arts, current events, your latest project.   One point for T: ___

d. Philosophy, ideals.   One point for P: ___

43. Which of the following best describes your disposition?

a. Sensuous, warm and comfortable.   One point for G: ___

b. Friendly, open and practical.   One point for A: ___

c. Artistic, lively and changeable.   One point for T: ___

d. Intellectual, cool and detached.   One point for P: ___

44. When you feel negative, you are most apt to become:

a. Weepy.   One point for G: ___

b. Irritable.   One point for A: ✓___

c. Depressed.   One point for T: ___

d. Neurotic.   One point for P: ___

45. Which of the following best describes your temper?

a. Quick-tempered but easily distracted   One point for G: ___
   from your anger by flattery or apologies.

b. Slow to get angry, but once you are,   One point for A: ___
   you stay mad for a while.

c. Quick-tempered over small matters,   One point for T: ___
   inclined to get depressed when irritated.

d. Slow to get angry and quick to get   One point for P: ✓___
   over it, once you have a chance to
   think things over.

Now add up your points for each type.
Total Score for Section 7:

G:___2___ A:___2___ T:_____ P:___1___

Scoring Instruction:

Go through your Total Scores for all seven sections and add them together. Write the total for all sections here:

G: ___28___ A: ___12___ T: ___8___ P: ___8___

Now look at your score. Your highest number indicates your body type.

If your highest number of answers is G, you are a Gonadal Type. Turn to Chapter 6 for the G-Type Weight Loss Program.

If your highest number of answers is A, you are an Adrenal Type. Turn to Chapter 7 for the A-Type Weight Loss Program.

If your highest number of answers is T, you are a Thyroid Type. Turn to Chapter 8 for the T-Type Weight Loss Program.

If your highest number of answers is P, you are a Pituitary Type. Turn to Chapter 9 for the P-Type Weight Loss Program.

SPECIAL INSTRUCTIONS IF YOU HAVE A TIE:

A tie indicates that your body type is well balanced. However, you do have a dominant gland which will determine your type. In this case you should use *only* your answers from Sections 1, 2, and 3, since appearance is more clearly indicative of body type than any of the other factors.

SPECIAL INSTRUCTIONS FOR GONADAL TYPES:

If your score indicates that you are a G-Type but your ovaries are no longer active (either because you have passed the menopause or because of surgery), you should consider yourself as being the body type with the *next* highest number of answers. However, if you are taking female sex hormones, you should still consider yourself G-Type, since the supplementary hormones you are taking take the place of your body's natural hormones and this enables you to retain the metabolism of a G-Type.

THE BODY TYPE CHECK LIST FOR MEN

SECTION 1: BODY SHAPE AND APPEARANCE

1. Look at yourself straight on in the mirror, focusing on the overall outline and shape of your body.

   a. My body is square and sturdy and looks as if I played football. (See Figure 9, page 73.)

   Two points for A: __

   b. My body is long-limbed and looks as if I played basketball. (See Figure 11, page 75.)

   Two points for T: __

   c. My body is boyish and looks much as it did when I was fourteen. (See Figure 13, page 77.)

   Two points for P: __

2. Now turn sideways to the mirror and focus on the line of your back.

   a. My back is slightly "swayed" and my rear end appears slightly rounded. (See Figure 10, page 74.)

   Two points for A: __

   b. My back is straight and I have practically no rear end. (See Figure 12, page 76.)

   Two points for T: __

   c. My back is curved and my head comes forward from my neck. (See Figure 14, page 78.)

   Two points for P: __

3. Next, focus on your head—its shape and its relation to your body size.

   a. My head is squarish and I have a square or round face.

   Two points for A: __

   b. My head is long and I have a slender face.

   Two points for T: __

   c. My head is round and slightly large for my body size.

   Two points for P: __

4. Examine your hands and feet. They are:

a. Square, with short fingers and toes.   Two points for A: ___

b. Long, with tapering fingers and toes.   Two points for T: ___

c. Small, delicate.   Two points for P: ___

5. Focus on your teeth. They are:

a. Large, slightly yellowish.   Two points for A: ___

b. Small, white, even.   Two points for T: ___

c. Large, especially front center.   Two points for P: ___

6. Look at the shape of your mouth. It is:

a. Full.   Two points for A: ___

b. Wide, mobile.   Two points for T: ___

c. Curved, well-shaped.   Two points for P: ___

7. Look at your skin. It is:

a. Oily, slightly coarse, ruddy   Two points for A: ___

b. Smooth, of normal oiliness.   Two points for T: ___

c. Dry, delicate.   Two points for P: ___

8. Finally, think back to when you were at your ideal weight, or try to imagine how you would look at your normal weight based on what you have already observed about your present shape. At your ideal weight you would be:

a. Substantial and strong looking.   Two points for A: ___

b. Rangy and fine-boned.   Two points for T: ___

c. Boyish and slender.   Two points for P: ___

Now add up your points for each type.
Total Score for Section 1:

A:_____ T:_____ P:_____

SECTION 2: FAT DISTRIBUTION

9. Look at yourself in the mirror, focusing on your excess weight. Where is *most* of your fat?

a. Across the stomach in a "beer   Two points for A: ___
belly," or across the upper back.

b. Around the middle in a "roll."   Two points for T: ___

c. All over, no single location.   Two points for P: ___

10. Look at yourself from the back, or ask your friend to look. Do you have more fat:

a. Across the upper back.   Two points for A: ___

b. Around the waist in "love handles."   Two points for T: ___

c. All over—not more above or below.   Two points for P: ___

11. Focus on your hands and feet. Do
they have an accumulation of fat?

a. Yes, bones aren't clearly outlined.   One point for A: ___

and   One point for P: ___

b. No, bones are cleary outlined.   One point for T: ___

Now add up your points for each type.
Total Score for Part 2:

A:_____ T:_____ P:_____

SECTION 3: FOOD PREFERENCES

12. Of the following foods, which do you
love the most?

a. Steak, salty foods.   One point for A: ___

b. Bread, sweets.   One point for T: ___

c. Dairy products.   One point for P: ___

13. At a party, which of these foods
would you find hardest to resist?

a. The hot dogs, salami or peanuts.   One point for A: ___

b. The cakes or candies.   One point for T: ___

c. The ice cream or frozen yogurt.   One point for P: ___

14. How much coffee, tea or cola do you
   drink each day?
a. Three or four cups.   One point for A: ___

b. Five cups or more.   One point for T: ___

c. None, or one or two cups.   One point for P: ___

15. Which of the following would you
   prefer for breakfast?
a. Bacon and eggs.   One point for A: ___

b. Toast and jam.   One point for T: ___

c. Fruit and yogurt.   One point for P: ___

16. Ideally, when would you like to have
   your biggest meal?
a. Late in the day.   One point for A: ___

b. Early in the day.   One point for T: ___

d. Prefer no big meal, just lots of snacks. One point for P: ___

___

Now add up your points for each type.
Total Score for Section 3:
A:_____ T:_____ P:_____

SECTION 4: ENERGY PATTERNS

17. Ideally, how many hours do you sleep each night?

a. 4-6 hours.   One point for A: ___

b. 5-6 hours in good periods, 9-10 hours when tired.   One point for T: ___

c. 7-8 hours.   One point for P: ___

18. When does your highest-energy period occur?

a. Energetic all day.   One point for A: ___

b. Following meals, especially breakfast and dinner.   One point for T: ___

c. First thing in the morning.   One point for P: ___

19. Do you have trouble sleeping at night?

a. Often.   One point for A: ___

b. Occasionally, but only for one night at a time.   One point for T: ___

c. Occasionally, but when I do it happens every night for a while.   One point for P: ___

Now add up your points for each type.
Total Score for Section 4:

A:_____ T:_____ P:_____

SECTION 5: BODILY RESPONSES

20. How much do you perspire?
    a. Quite a bit, even at rest.   One point for A: ___

    b. Variably. Very lightly when slim,   One point for T: ___
       more when heavy.
    c. Lightly.   One point for P: ___

21. Are you prone to colds and allergies?
    a. No, almost never.   One point for A: ___

    b. Yes, quite a bit.   One point for T: ___

       and   One point for P: ___

22. Are you prone to upset stomach or
    diarrhea?
    a. Rarely.   One point for A: ___

    b. Yes.   One point for T: ___

       and   One point for P: ___

23. Are you prone to headaches?
    a. Rarely.   One point for A: ___

    b. Occasionally.   One point for T: ___

    c. Yes, quite a bit.   One point for P: ___

24. Do your hands and feet feel cold at night?

a. Rarely.   One point for A: ___

b. Often.   One point for T: ___

c. No.   One point for P: ___

25. When you are ill, which parts of your body are most likely to ache?

a. Lower back.   One point for A: ___

b. Neck and shoulders.   One point for T: ___

c. Knees.   One point for P: ___

26. Which of your senses is the most important to you—that is, the one you use most in making up your mind about the qualities of an object?

a. Hearing.   One point for A: ___

b. Taste/smell.   One point for T: ___

c. Sight.   One point for P: ___

27. Which of your senses is the least important to you—that is, the one you weigh the least in judging an object?

a. Taste/smell.   One point for A: ___

b. Hearing.   One point for T: ___

c. Touch.   One point for P: ___

28. Ideally, how often would you like to
make love?

a. Three times a week or more.   One point for A: ___

b. In spurts. A lot for a while, then not   One point for T: ___
at all for a while.

c. Once a week or less.   One point for P: ___

Now add up your points for each type.
Total Score for Section 5:

A:_____ T:_____ P:_____

SECTION 6: PERSONALITY TRAITS

29. Is it easy for you to laugh at yourself?
(Be honest, now!)

a. No.   One point for A: ___

b. Yes.   One point for T: ___

c. Usually—not when I'm tired.   One point for P: ___

30. Which of these subjects do you most
enjoy discussing or thinking about?

a. Business, money, practical things   One point for A: ___

b. My latest project—it varies.   One point for T: ___

c. Philosophy, the arts.   One point for P: ___

31. Which of the following best describes your disposition?

a. Friendly, open and practical.   One point for A: ___

b. Artistic, lively and changeable.   One point for T: ___

c. Intellectual, cool and detached.   One point for P: ___

32. When you feel negative, you are most apt to become:

a. Irritable.   One point for A: ___

b. Depressed.   One point for T: ___

c. Neurotic.   One point for P: ___

33. Which of the following best describes your temper?

a. Slow to get angry, but once I am, I stay mad for a while.   One point for A: ___

b. Quick-tempered over small matters, inclined to get depressed when irritated.   One point for T: ___

c. Slow to get angry and quick to get over it, once I have a chance to think things over.   One point for P: ___

Now add up your points for each type.
Total Score for Section 6:

A:_____ T:_____ P:_____

Scoring Instruction:
    Go through your Total Scores for all six sections and add them together. Write the total for all sections here:

A:_____ T:_____ P:_____

Now look at your score. Your highest number indicates your body type.

If your highest number of answers is A, you are an Adrenal Type. Turn to Chapter 7 for the A-Type Weight Loss Program.

If your highest number of answers is T, you are a Thyroid Type. Turn to Chapter 8 for the T-Type Weight Loss Program.

If your highest number of answers is P, you are a Pituitary Type. Turn to Chapter 9 for the P-Type Weight Loss Program.

SPECIAL INSTRUCTIONS IF YOU HAVE A TIE:

A tie indicates that your body type is well balanced. However, you do have a dominant gland which will determine your type. In this case you should use *only* your answers from Sections 1, 2, and 3, since appearance is more clearly indicative of body type than any of the other factors.

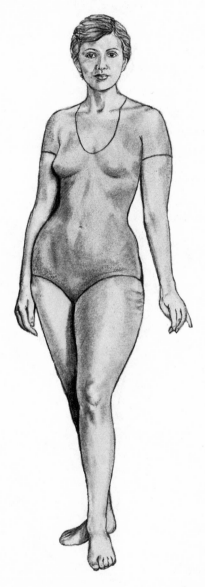

FIGURE 1: The **G-type** woman front view. Note difference in size between upper and lower body, small waist, "saddle bags" on outer thighs.

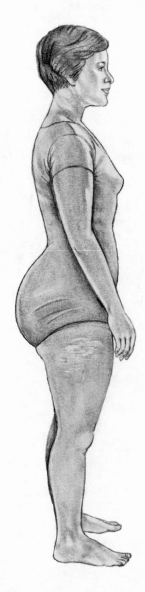

FIGURE 2: The **G-type** woman in profile. Note large rear end, relatively flat stomach, sway-back line of back.

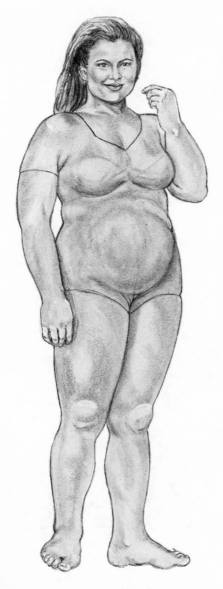

FIGURE 3: The **A-type** woman front view. Note straight, sturdy line of body, squarish or round face, large breasts.

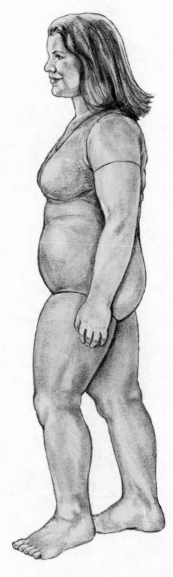

FIGURE 4: The **A-type** woman in profile. Note straight back, "tucked-under" rear end, pot belly, thickness in arms and legs all the way down.

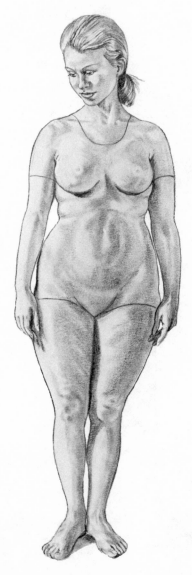

FIGURE 5: The **T-Type** woman front view. Note heavy thighs, tapering legs, delicate feet, hands, and head. In spite of fat, waist remains distinct.

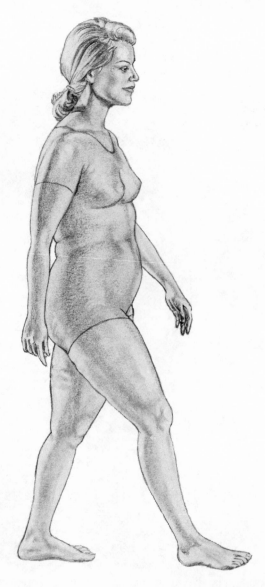

FIGURE 6: The **T-type** woman in profile. Note rounded, but not pronounced, rear end, round shoulders, tummy fat mostly below the navel.

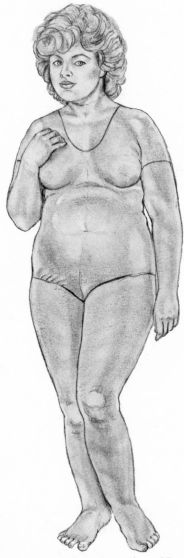

FIGURE 7: The **P-type** woman front view. Note childlike or "undeveloped" look, appearance of baby fat, small breasts, relatively large head.

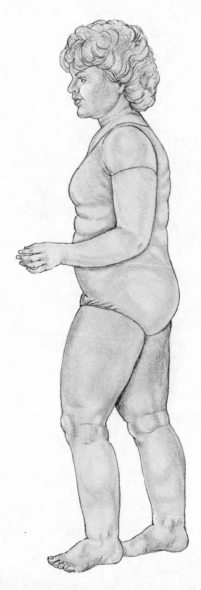

FIGURE 8: The **P-type** woman in profile. Note rounded shoulders, small rear, pudgy knees, childlike "tummy."

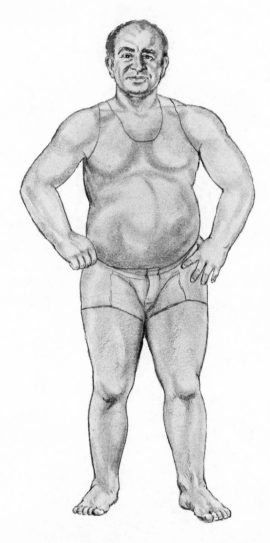

FIGURE 9: The **A-type** man front view. Note broad chest, thickened waist, and straight, thick thighs. The build is straight and full from mid-chest to knees.

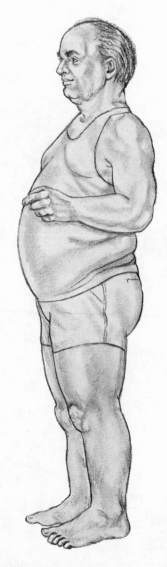

FIGURE 10: The **A-type** man in profile. Note classic pot belly, rounded rear end, thick neck, bulky muscles.

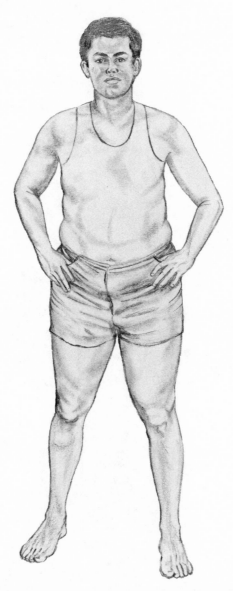

FIGURE 11: The **T-type** man front view. Note long limbs, fat accumulation in upper arms and thighs, tummy fat arranged in "rolls."

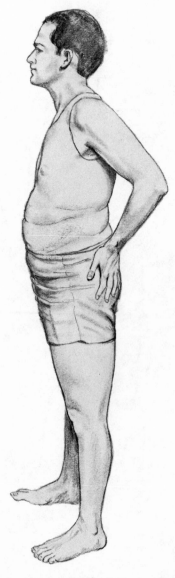

FIGURE 12: The **T-type** man in profile. Note straight back, flat rear, delicate neck.

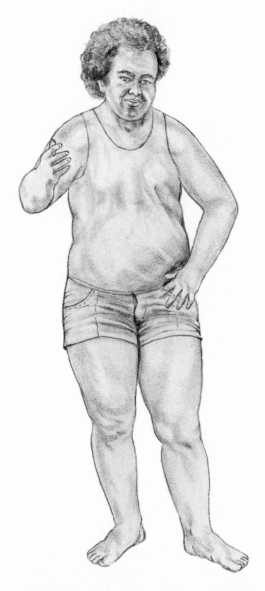

FIGURE 13: The **P-type** man front view. Note boyish, relatively un-developed look, sloping shoulders, concave chest.

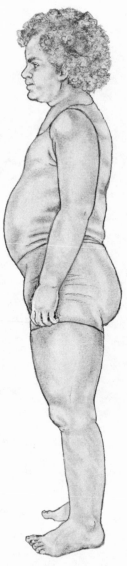

FIGURE 14: The **P-type** man in profile. Note contrast to A-type: higher, more rounded pot belly; softer, less "beefy" fat; more child-like head; less developed muscles.

6

THE GONADAL BODY TYPE WEIGHT LOSS PROGRAM

THE BASIC STRATEGY FOR G-TYPES

The key to weight loss for you as a gonadal type is to simultaneously decrease stimulation to your gonads and increase it to your thyroid and pituitary. All of the problems you encounter in losing weight can be traced directly to the excessive dominance of the gonads on the one hand and the weakness in thyroid and pituitary function on the other.

The best way to accomplish this is to cut out red meat, creamy and fatty foods. While on your Basic Weight Loss Program do not eat any red meat *at all*. Even the lighter proteins found in chicken, fish and eggs are reduced. All creamy, buttery dishes are also completely eliminated. For the necessary fat in your diet you are allowed a small amount of vegetable oil.

ELIMINATE SPICES (HERBS ARE OK)

On the G-Type Weight Loss Program spices are eliminated in favor of non-stimulating herbs. Many popular diets urge dieters to spice up their foods, since spices add variety and have no calories. This is acceptable for other body types, but not for G-types. The idea is to rest the sex glands, not to continue overstimulating them. Herbs such as dill, parsley, basil, tarragon, and thyme are fine. You can use a tiny bit of salt (see "Recipes for G-Types"), but go easy.

CONCENTRATE ON
CHICKEN, FISH AND
DAIRY FOODS

Since red meat is eliminated, for protein eat plenty of chicken, fish and light dairy products instead of red meat. Yogurt and cottage cheese are excellent foods for you, not only for their protein but for the stimulation they give to the pituitary gland. I also have given you a glass of nonfat milk at both lunch and dinner. The protein in the milk is light and nonstimulating to the gonads, but gives you enough staying power so you will not feel hungry in the afternoon or evening.

TAKE CARBOHYDRATES
IN MODERATION, EVEN
A LITTLE CAFFEINE

Your system benefits from a moderate intake of carbohydrates, partially from whole grains, partially from ordinary refined grains. Eat lots of fruit. Fruit is an excellent food for you; it provides natural stimulation to the thyroid gland.

You may have a small amount of caffeine (coffee or tea) as well, with a little sugar in the morning. Allowing even ½ teaspoon of sugar is unusual for a diet, but in your case it is an effective part of the strategy of thyroid and pituitary stimulation.

THE TOTAL STRATEGY

Summarizing your total dieting strategy: no red meat, a minimum of fat and oil, lots of fruit and fresh vegetables, plenty of light dairy products, a small amount of sugar and caffeine, a moderate amount of carbohydrates, mostly from whole grains, and no stimulating spices.

The results for you will be a lighter, less sluggish metabolism, more energy, faster weight loss than you've ever experienced, and (especially during your Last Five Pounds Diet) a dramatic loss of the cellulite (the wrinkly fat commonly found on hips, thighs, buttocks, or upper arms) that virtually all G-types over the age of fifteen are so prone to acquire.

THE G-TYPE MEAL SCHEDULE

EAT VERY LIGHTLY IN THE MORNING

Most important is that you start the day with a *very* light breakfast. What works for G-Types is to eat for breakfast only a small piece of fruit and a cup of coffee or tea (either regular tea or Red Clover Tea).

Many successful, slender G-types give credit to their light breakfasts for losing and keeping off their fat. If they start the day with a heavy meal, they eat all day long. Starting with a light breakfast keeps them light all day.

The gonads are more active at night than in the early hours of the day, which means that your metabolism handles food better later in the day than early.

EAT LIGHTLY AT LUNCH

Your lunch is also fairly light, so that your body continues on a fat-burning metabolism throughout the afternoon. My patients tell me how well it works for them to stay with light food throughout the day. Not only is weight loss faster, they actually feel lighter and get more accomplished than if they burden themselves with a heavy meal at lunchtime.

DINNER IS SUBSTANTIAL

Your most substantial meal comes in the evening. This is not only most effective in terms of burning fat, it will also help you avoid snacking at night, a time when many G-types respond to the increased activity of the dominant gland with what I call "sensual" eating (eating for sensual enjoyment, as opposed to eating for stimulation).

OBSERVE THE
INTERVALS BETWEEN
MEALS

You *must* observe the intervals which I specify between meals. These are four hours between breakfast and lunch and five hours between lunch and dinner on the Basic Weight Loss Diet, and five hours between breakfast and lunch and six between lunch and dinner on the Last Five Pounds Diet. Even though the G-type breakfast is very light, and lunch not very heavy either, the intervals remain important. It is during these periods that the body burns fat.

YOUR DANGER
PERIODS

You have two danger periods for snacking: late morning and late evening. These are times when your metabolism is at a low ebb. The morning "low" is due to a lessening of thyroidal activity following the thyroid-stimulating breakfast, and the evening "low" relates to increased late-evening activity of the gonads, which produces an impulse towards sensual eating.

YOUR BEST SNACK

However, it is not physically necessary for you to eat anything at all at either of these times. Your thyroid gland is strong and will revive after a short "low" in the morning without any intervention.

A G-type patient once commented that she'd been very apt to snack in the late morning once she'd given up her former giant breakfasts. She was experiencing a momentary thyroidal lag. When she tried sitting down for ten minutes with a cup of Red Clover Tea, instead of having a snack, she found that at the end of the ten minutes she felt good again, and the desire to snack had passed of its own accord.

If you absolutely must have a more substantial snack, take a small portion of fruit—for example, a few grapes or a couple of strawberries. They will stimulate your thyroid gently and get you through to the next meal. A small amount of fruit is also the snack of choice if you find yourself doing "sensual eating" late at night. If this is a pattern for you, you may save your dinner fruit and eat it instead later in the evening.

THE G-TYPE HERBAL HELP: RED CLOVER TEA

Red Clover Tea is a "must" for G-type weight loss—it makes dieting not only much easier but much more efficient as well. Red Clover is a tea which is traditionally used to ease menstrual problems, and your overstimulated and overtired gonads benefit tremendously from its restorative powers. You make it like this: Bring water to a full boil and add a teaspoon of Red Clover Tops for every cup of tea you want. Allow to steep for five minutes, strain and serve. You may use a half teaspoon of honey or sugar with your tea if you wish. Red Clover Tops are available in most health food stores.

RULES FOR G-TYPE DIETING

In the following pages are both general guidelines for G-type dieting (a complete list of exactly what you are to eat for each meal, both for the Basic Weight Loss Diet and the Last Five Pounds Diet) and a week of sample menus for each of the diets. You may use the sample menus or substitute your own, as long as you use only the permitted foods and follow the guidelines exactly.

You may substitute freely *within the boundaries allowed for each meal,* but may not rearrange the food among meals. Poultry and fish may only be broiled, grilled or baked (see guidelines for each meal). Vegetables may be steamed, boiled in a small amount of water, or sauteed in the permitted vegetable oil only. Seasonal fruit may be substituted for the suggested fruit at any meal. Poultry is to be eaten without skin. *Do not omit anything; every food is there for a reason.*

THE COMPLETE
GONADAL-TYPE
WEIGHT LOSS
PROGRAM

Begin with one week of the Basic G-Type Weight Loss Diet. How long you follow it depends on how much weight you want to lose.

TO LOSE FIFTEEN POUNDS OR MORE: Follow the Basic G-Type Weight Loss Diet for three weeks and then the G-Type Last Five Pounds Diet for a week. Then go back to the G-Type Basic Weight Loss diet, changing to the Last Five Pounds Diet every fourth week for as long as needed. When you are within five pounds of your ideal weight, change to the Last Five Pounds Diet and finish your weight loss with it.

TO LOSE FIVE TO FIFTEEN POUNDS: Follow the G-Type Basic Weight Loss diet for two weeks, then the G-Type Last Five Pounds Diet for a week (or less, if you reach your ideal weight before the end of the final week).

TO LOSE FIVE POUNDS OR LESS: Follow the G-Type Basic Weight Loss Diet for one week, then the G-Type Last Five Pounds Diet for a week (or less).

WHEN YOU REACH YOUR IDEAL WEIGHT: Change to the Health and Weight Maintenance Program for G-types.

Dishes which are marked with an asterisk are those for which a recipe is provided in Appendix 1.

THE BASIC
G-TYPE
WEIGHT LOSS
DIET:
GENERAL
GUIDELINES

BREAKFAST

One small piece of fruit (choice of 1 apple or: 2 apricots, ½ banana, 1 cup of berries, ¼ cantaloupe, 10 cherries, 2 fresh figs, ½ mango, 1 nectarine, 1 peach, 1 pear, ½ cup of fresh pineapple, 2 plums, 1 cup of strawberries or 1 cup of watermelon)

Coffee, tea or Red Clover Tea (with ½ teaspoon of sugar or honey if desired)

WAIT FOUR HOURS

LUNCH

Large green salad of any combination of lettuce, cucumber, mushrooms, celery, sprouts, radishes, bell pepper, tomato and onion

1 teaspoon of any *clear* diet dressing (not creamy or spicy)

Choice of ½ cup of beets, carrots, cauliflower, peas, pumpkin, squash or turnip

2 ounces of lowfat hard cheese OR 1 cup of yogurt OR 1 cup of lowfat cottage cheese OR 1 egg (soft or hard-boiled, or fried in 1 teaspoon of vegetable oil only)

1 slice of whole-grain bread (rye bread is recommended), without butter

1 glass of skim milk

1 piece of fruit, from the same choices as offered at breakfast

Coffee, tea or Red Clover Tea (with ½ teaspoon of sugar or honey if desired)

WAIT FIVE HOURS

DINNER

Choice of 4 ounces of chicken OR 4 ounces of turkey OR 4 ounces of fish OR 2 eggs. (The eggs may be soft or hard-boiled, or fried in 1 teaspoon of vegetable oil. You should not have eggs if you had an egg for lunch.)

1 teaspoon of vegetable oil may be used in preparation of the poultry or fish, on the vegetables, or to cook your eggs

Steamed vegetables, your choice, as much as you like

Choice of 1 slice of whole-grain bread OR ½ cup of bulghur wheat OR ½ cup of brown rice OR ½ cup of millet—no butter

1 piece of fruit, from the same choices as breakfast

1 glass of skim milk

Red Clover Tea (with ½ teaspoon of sugar or honey if desired)

THE BASIC
G-TYPE WEIGHT
LOSS DIET: A
WEEK OF SAMPLE
MENUS

MONDAY

BREAKFAST: 1 large nectarine (or other fruit in season)
Coffee, tea or Red Clover Tea (sugar or honey if
desired)

LUNCH: Large green salad with clear diet dressing*
1 cup of plain yogurt
1 slice of rye toast
1 plum (or other fruit in season)
1 glass of skim milk
Hot tea (sugar or honey if desired)

DINNER: Stir-fried Chicken* (or substitute your own chicken
recipe, as long as the chicken is cooked without
skin and without additional fat or oil)
½ cup of white rice
Cucumber salad dressed with 1 tablespoon of
yogurt
1 glass of skim milk
1 peach (or other fruit in season)
Red Clover Tea (sugar or honey if desired)

TUESDAY

BREAKFAST: ½ mango (or other fruit in season)
Coffee, tea or Red Clover Tea (sugar or honey if
desired)

LUNCH: Large green salad with clear diet dressing*
1 hard-boiled egg
1 slice of whole-wheat toast
1 glass of skim milk

½ papaya (or other fruit in season)
Iced tea (regular or Red Clover, sugar or honey if
    desired)

DINNER: 4 ounces of Chicken Salad with Yogurt* (or use
    your own chicken recipe, prepared without
    skin or added oil)
Steamed spinach, as much as you like
2 pieces of rye Krispbread
1 cup of strawberries (or other fruit in season)
1 glass of skim milk
Red Clover Tea (sugar or honey if desired)

WEDNESDAY

BREAKFAST: 2 plums (or other fruit in season)
Coffee, tea or Red Clover Tea (sugar or honey if
    desired)

LUNCH: 2 ounces of lowfat string cheese
1 slice of whole-grain bread
Large green salad with clear diet dressing*
1 glass of skim milk
1 apple (or other fruit in season)
Coffee (sugar or honey if desired)

DINNER: Greek-Style Eggs* (or use your own egg recipe,
    prepared with teaspoon of vegetable oil only)
Steamed zucchini and string beans
1 cup of green grapes (or other fruit in season)
1 glass of skim milk
Red Clover Tea (sugar or honey if desired)

THURSDAY

BREAKFAST: ½ banana (or other fruit in season)
Coffee, tea or Red Clover Tea (sugar or honey if
    desired)

LUNCH: 1 cup of lowfat cottage cheese
Large green salad with clear diet dressing*

2 pieces of rye Krispbread
½ mango (or other fruit in season)
1 glass of skim milk
Tea (regular or Red Clover, sugar or honey if desired)

DINNER: Marinated Fish with Vegetables* (or use your own fish recipe, using no breading and 1 teaspoon of vegetable oil only)
½ cup cole slaw (made with cabbage and 1 teaspoon diet mayonnaise)
½ cup of bulghur wheat*
1 cup of fresh cherries (or other fruit in season)
1 glass of skim milk
Red Clover Tea (sugar or honey if desired)

FRIDAY

BREAKFAST: 2 apricots (or other fruit in season)
Coffee, tea or Red Clover Tea (sugar or honey if desired)

LUNCH: 1 cup of yogurt
1 cup of strawberries (or other fruit in season)
Large green salad with clear diet dressing*
1 slice of rye toast
Tea (regular or Red Clover, sugar or honey if desired)

DINNER: Lemon Chicken Kabobs* (or use your own chicken recipe, prepared without skin or added oil)
½ cup of millet*
1 apple (or other fruit in season)
1 glass of skim milk
Red Clover Tea (sugar or honey if desired)

SATURDAY

BREAKFAST: ½ cantaloupe (or other fruit in season)
Coffee, tea or Red Clover Tea (sugar or honey if desired)

LUNCH: 1 hard-boiled egg
1 slice of whole-grain toast
Large green salad with clear diet dressing*
1 glass of skim milk
½ banana (or other fruit in season)
Tea (regular or Red Clover, sugar or honey if desired)

DINNER: Salmon Steak Florentine* (or use your own fish recipe, prepared without breading or additional oil)
½ cup of rice
1 pear (or other fruit in season)
1 glass of skim milk
Red Clover Tea (sugar or honey if desired)

SUNDAY

BREAKFAST: 1 cup of unsweetened applesauce (or other fruit in season)
Coffee, Tea or Red Clover Tea

LUNCH: 2 ounces of hard cheese
1 slice of rye toast
Large green salad with clear diet dressing*
1 glass of skim milk
2 tangerines (or other fruit in season)
Coffee (sugar or honey if desired)

DINNER: Stir-Fried Fish Fillets* (or use your own fish recipe, prepared without breading or additional oil)
½ cup of bulghur wheat*
2 fresh figs (or other fruit in season)
1 glass of skim milk
Red Clover Tea (sugar or honey if desired)

THE G-TYPE LAST FIVE POUNDS DIET

Remember, do not begin this diet until you have followed the Basic G-Type Weight Loss Diet for *at least* a week. The sequence of diets (see page 84) is vital not only for losing weight, but for bringing your metabolism into balance so that you can stay at your ideal weight.

The G-Type Last Five Pounds Diet is a special diet. It is designed for breaking the "plateaus" that occur regularly in the course of losing weight, as well as for getting off the last five pounds that are particularly difficult to lose for everyone. It contains about 1000 calories per day, 200 less than the G-Type Basic Weight Loss Diet. If you were to begin the Last Five Pounds Diet immediately, right at the start of your dieting program, you would undoubtedly feel quite hungry. However, since you have already followed the G-Type Basic Weight Loss Program for at least a week, your metabolism has been strengthened and brought into improved balance. A healthier and more balanced body is far less likely to experience excessive hunger while dieting.

Be aware that the interval between meals is longer on the Last Five Pounds Diet than on the Basic Weight Loss Diet. Again, the more balanced state of your metabolism will allow you to observe the longer interval comfortably.

The Last Five Pounds Diet is only to be followed for a week at a time. If, at the end of a week, you have not yet reached your ideal weight, change back to the G-Type Basic Weight Loss Diet for one, two or three more weeks, as necessary, until you are within five pounds of your ideal weight. Use the Last Five Pounds Diet for these last, stubborn pounds. Then, when you are at your ideal weight, change to the G-Type Health and Weight Maintenance Diet (see page 99 for the complete program).

The days you spend on the G-Type Last Five Pounds Diet are the most important days of your diet. These are the days when your body is most active in removing fat and, especially, cellulite.

The loss of cellulite you will be experiencing indicates that your body is reaching a healthy state of equilibrium among the glands. Without this state of equilibrium, you always have the potential for becoming overweight again. The loss of cellulite tells you that your body is acquiring the ability to maintain itself at its ideal weight.

THE LAST FIVE POUNDS DIET: GENERAL GUIDELINES

BREAKFAST

1 piece of fruit (choice of: 1 apple, 2 apricots, ½ banana, 1 cup of berries, ¼ cantaloupe, 10 cherries, 2 fresh figs, ½ mango, 1 nectarine, 1 peach, 1 pear, ½ cup of fresh pineapple, 2 plums, 1 cup of strawberries or 1 cup of watermelon)

Coffee, tea or Red Clover Tea (with ½ teaspoon sugar or honey, if desired)

WAIT FIVE HOURS

LUNCH

3 ounces lowfat hard cheese (such as Parmesan or Romano) or 3 ounces of lowfat soft cheese (such as lowfat string cheese or diet American cheese.)

1 slice of whole-grain bread

1 teaspoon of butter or diet mayonnaise

1 piece of fruit (same choices as breakfast)

G-Type Vegetable Soup,* as much as you like

Red Clover Tea (with ½ teaspoon of sugar or honey, if desired)

WAIT SIX HOURS

DINNER

1 cup of plain yogurt OR 4 ounces of lowfat cheese OR 2 eggs OR 1 egg and 2 ounces of lowfat cheese

G-Type Vegetable Soup,* as much as you like

1 teaspoon of vegetable oil or butter (you may cook your egg in this, or use it on your bread or rice)

½ cup of white rice OR 1 slice of whole-grain bread

1 piece of fruit (same choices as breakfast)

Red Clover Tea (with ½ teaspoon of sugar or honey, if desired)

THE G-TYPE LAST FIVE POUNDS DIET: A WEEK OF SAMPLE MENUS

MONDAY

BREAKFAST: Your choice of fruit—1 small piece
Coffee, tea or Red Clover Tea (sugar or honey if desired)

LUNCH: G-Type Vegetable Soup* (as much as you like)
1 slice of whole-grain bread
1 teaspoon of butter
2 ounces of Parmesan cheese
Your choice of fruit—1 small piece
Red Clover Tea (sugar or honey if desired)

DINNER: 1 cup of yogurt
G-Type Vegetable Soup* (as much as you like)
½ cup of rice
1 teaspoon of butter
Your choice of fruit—1 small piece
Red Clover Tea (sugar or honey if desired)

TUESDAY

BREAKFAST: Your choice of fruit—1 small piece
Coffee, tea or Red Clover Tea (sugar or honey if desired)

LUNCH: G-Type Vegetable Soup* (as much as you like)
1 slice of whole-grain bread
1 teaspoon of butter
3 ounces of string cheese
Your choice of fruit—1 small piece
Red Clover Tea (sugar or honey if desired)

DINNER: Eggs Mornay*
           G-Type Vegetable Soup* (as much as you like)
           1 slice of whole-grain bread
           1 teaspoon of butter
           Your choice of fruit—1 small piece
           Red Clover Tea (sugar or honey if desired)

WEDNESDAY

BREAKFAST: Your choice of fruit—1 small piece
           Coffee, tea or Red Clover Tea (sugar or honey if
              desired)

LUNCH: G-Type Vegetable Soup* (as much as you like)
           1 slice of whole-grain bread
           1 teaspoon of butter
           2 ounces of Parmesan cheese
           Your choice of fruit—1 small piece
           Red Clover Tea (sugar or honey if desired)

DINNER: Herb Omelette*
           G-Type Vegetable Soup* (as much as you like)
           ½ cup of rice
           1 teaspoon of butter
           Your choice of fruit—1 small piece
           Red Clover Tea (sugar or honey if desired)

THURSDAY

BREAKFAST: Your choice of fruit—1 small piece
           Coffee, tea or Red Clover Tea
              (sugar or honey if desired)

LUNCH: G-Type Vegetable Soup* (as much as you like)
           1 slice of whole-grain bread
           1 teaspoon of butter
           2 ounces of Romano cheese
           Your choice of fruit—1 small piece
           Red Clover Tea (sugar or honey if desired)

DINNER: 1 cup of plain yogurt
            G-Type Vegetable Soup* (as much as you like)
            1 slice of whole-grain bread
            1 teaspoon of butter
            Your choice of fruit—1 small piece
            Red Clover Tea (sugar or honey if desired)

FRIDAY

BREAKFAST: Your choice of fruit—1 small piece
            Coffee, tea or Red Clover Tea
              (sugar or honey if desired)

LUNCH: G-Type Vegetable Soup* (as much as you like)
            1 slice of whole-grain bread
            1 teaspoon of butter
            3 ounces of lowfat string cheese
            Your choice of fruit—1 small piece
            Red Clover Tea (sugar or honey if desired)

DINNER: 2 Poached Eggs
            G-Type Vegetable Soup* (as much as you like)
            ½ cup of rice
            1 teaspoon of butter
            Your choice of fruit—1 small piece
            Red Clover Tea (sugar or honey if desired)

SATURDAY

BREAKFAST: Your choice of fruit—1 small piece
            Coffee, tea or Red Clover Tea
              (sugar or honey if desired)

LUNCH: G-Type Vegetable Soup* (as much as you like)
            1 slice of whole-grain bread
            1 teaspoon of butter
            3 ounces of diet American cheese
            Your choice of fruit—1 small piece
            Red Clover Tea (sugar or honey if desired)

DINNER: Spaghetti with Cheese*
G-Type Vegetable Soup* (as much as you like)
Your choice of fruit—1 small piece
Red Clover Tea (sugar or honey if desired)

SUNDAY

BREAKFAST: Your choice of fruit—1 small piece
Coffee, tea or Red Clover Tea
(sugar or honey if desired)

LUNCH: G-Type Vegetable Soup* (as much as you like)
1 slice of whole-grain bread
1 teaspoon of butter
3 ounces of lowfat string cheese
Your choice of fruit—1 small piece
Red Clover Tea (sugar or honey if desired)

DINNER: 1 cup of plain yogurt
G-Type Vegetable Soup* (as much as you like)
½ cup of rice
1 teaspoon of butter
Your choice of fruit—1 small piece
Red Clover Tea (sugar or honey if desired)

THE G-TYPE HEALTH AND WEIGHT MAINTENANCE PROGRAM

The surest formula for keeping the ideal weight you've achieved through your Gonadal Type Weight Loss Program is to have a continuing awareness of your body type and its special needs. Your G-Type Diet has brought about a state of balance in your metabolism; the G-Type Health and Weight Maintenance Program is designed to make it easy for you to *maintain* that balance, and to keep your ideal weight.

"PLENTY," "MODERATION" AND "RARELY" FOODS

To make it as easy as possible for you to keep your body type requirements in mind, your program includes a *short, simple* set of guidelines for your body type. You need only keep in mind: 1) your Plenty Foods (foods you can always eat, which will always be good for you); 2) your Moderation Foods (foods you can eat as long as you don't overdo them; and 3) your Rarely Foods (ones you should save for special occasions only, because eating them will tend to revive your old cravings and make it harder for you to keep to your guidelines).

Continue to use your Herbal Tea and your Vegetable Soup. They will continue to strengthen your metabolism and are the best possible means for you to maintain the healthy balance you have achieved.

IF YOU FORGET THE GUIDELINES AND GAIN WEIGHT

If you stay with your guidelines you will not find yourself putting on weight. But if you let your guidelines go for a while (for instance, during a holiday season or on a vacation) and you find yourself three to five pounds above your ideal weight, then go back to your original G-Type Weight Loss Program. With five extra pounds, you will need only a week of the G-Type Basic Weight Loss Diet and a weekend of the G-Type Last Five Pounds Diet to be right back at your perfect weight. It'll be all but painless, since you'll have going for you the fundamentally balanced, healthy state that you achieved on the Body Type Program.

THE G-TYPE HEALTH AND WEIGHT MAINTENANCE PROGRAM: GENERAL GUIDELINES

1. YOUR PLENTY FOODS:
Fruit
Fresh vegetables
Whole grains
Yogurt
Cottage cheese
Red Clover Tea

2. YOUR MODERATION FOODS:
Poultry
Fish
Skim milk
Light cheese
Vegetable oils
Light desserts
Coffee or tea

3. YOUR RARELY FOODS:
Red meat
Spices
Cream, sour cream, ice cream
Butter
Rich desserts

4. YOUR IDEAL EATING SCHEDULE:
A very light breakfast—or even no breakfast at all

A light lunch: salad and a sandwich

Your main meal at night

Watch out for evening and late morning snacking!

BREAKFAST

A large piece of fruit (with ½ cup of plain yogurt on very busy days) OR 1 cup of whole-grain cereal with skim milk

Coffee, tea or Red Clover Tea (with a teaspoon of sugar if you wish)

LUNCH

A large green salad with your favorite vegetables, and just a little dressing

A serving of lowfat cottage cheese or hard cheese

2 slices of whole-grain bread OR ½ cup of brown rice OR ½ cup of bulghur wheat OR ½ cup of millet

A glass of skim milk

A piece of fruit

Coffee, tea or Red Clover Tea (with a teaspoon of sugar if you wish)

DINNER

A serving of fish or poultry, OR 2 eggs. Eat meat once a week or less. Avoid pork and "variety meats" (salami, cold cuts, organ meats, poultry "rolls")

A serving of whole grain 4 times a week
(You may have refined grains 3 times a week if you wish)

Vegetables, cooked or raw, as much as you like

A glass of skim milk (optional)

A piece of fruit or a small, light dessert—but avoid creamy desserts and whipped cream

Coffee, tea or Red Clover Tea (with a teaspoon of sugar if you wish)

7

THE ADRENAL BODY TYPE WEIGHT LOSS PROGRAM

THE BASIC STRATEGY FOR A-TYPES

The strategy of the Adrenal Type Weight Loss Program has two principal features: it reduces stimulation to the adrenals and increases stimulation to the pituitary and thyroid. To rest the adrenals, you cut back on red meat, and so you get your protein from poultry and fish. You have the option of eating a small portion of red meat three times a week, but for best results eliminate it completely.

An A-type patient once complained bitterly about the reduction in red meat. Apparently he didn't feel he'd eaten unless he'd had an enormous steak. But after just two weeks on the diet his opinion changed. He said that maybe he'd always like steak, but he didn't *have* to eat it every night. He felt so much better on his diet, and besides, he said, "chicken and fish are really good!" It didn't hurt his cholesterol level any, either.

CARBOHYDRATES AND DAIRY PRODUCTS ARE FINE

While you are resting your adrenals you stimulate your thyroid with carbohydrates. You also stimulate your pituitary with an abundance of light dairy products—cottage cheese, yogurt, nonfat milk.

Your carbohydrates are divided between whole-grain and

refined. You eat whole-grain carbohydrates at breakfast and most lunches, but at dinner and a few lunches you eat a small amount of refined grains such as white flour and white rice.

My A-type patients are often surprised to find that I also allow a small dessert twice a week. This is unusual on a diet but, in your case, beneficial. Your metabolism is helped by the thyroidal stimulation which desserts afford.

CAFFEINE—OK FOR YOU

Caffeine, which is practically a "street drug" to the thyroid type, for you is beneficial in moderation. By stimulating your thyroid it adds "swirls and eddies" to the steady flow of the A-type metabolism. There is not much danger in your drinking too much caffeine, since it doesn't correspond to your innate craving structure.

EAT PLENTY OF VEGETABLES

A vegetarian diet is very suitable for your type of metabolism, although it is not *necessary* for you to be a vegetarian if you don't wish to. You must be careful to get enough protein from milk and cheese, but as long as you do this you can prosper on a vegetarian diet indefinitely.

THE TOTAL STRATEGY

To summarize your diet strategy: much less red meat; plenty of fresh vegetables, whole grains and fruit; protein mainly from poultry and fish; lots of light dairy products; a small amount of caffeine and sugar.

You'll enjoy, as a result, a lighter, more flexible metabolism; quicker weight loss than you've ever experienced due to the energy-burning qualities of the thyroid gland; and a greatly reduced appetite, since a large appetite is a result of overstimulated adrenals. Your cellulite on your stomach, back and upper arms will come off, especially during the weeks on the Last Five Pounds Diet. And you'll find that you'll feel more creative and thoughtful—an interesting side effect of the pituitary stimulation of the A-Type Diet.

THE A-TYPE MEAL SCHEDULE

EAT A LIGHT BREAKFAST

The key to your food timing is to eat a light breakfast. A-types are usually of the eggs-bacon-and-buttered-toast school, but this is the wrong way for someone with your type of metabolism to start the day. Cereal or dairy products start your day with mild thyroidal or pituitary stimulation, a much better strategy for you.

The adrenal glands become more and more active as the day progresses, with the afternoon and evening being their most active time. As they become more active, your appetite increases. Avoid stimulating them first thing in the morning.

KEEP IT LIGHT AT LUNCHTIME

Lunch should also be light: salad, dairy products or fish, and fruit. This will help keep your appetite under control later on; the longer you can wait for your main meal, the easier dieting will be.

DINNER IS YOUR MAIN MEAL

Your main meal comes at night, when your adrenals can handle it, though even dinner is not very heavy: poultry, fish, vegetables and fruit.

OBSERVE THE INTERVAL BETWEEN MEALS

You must be sure to keep to the full interval between meals: four hours between breakfast and lunch, six hours between lunch and dinner on the Basic Weight Loss Diet, five hours between breakfast and lunch and six hours between lunch and dinner on the Last Five Pounds Diet. It is during these hours that your body burns fat and rebalances itself metabolically; if you eat again too soon after a meal, you waste most of your dieting effort.

Losing weight, we now know, is not a simple matter of reducing calories. Losing weight means metabolizing fat, and you must give your body a chance to do it!

YOUR DANGER
PERIODS

Your danger period for snacking is late afternoon, because this is a period of tiredness after the work of the day that happens to correspond with the beginning of the adrenal gland's more active period. The combination of tiredness (which makes you want stimulation) and increased appetite means that you experience a double-danger period.

One A-type patient who was just starting on the A-Type Diet told me that he can go without breakfast and lunch without difficulty, but that when five o'clock comes around he finds himself snacking on all kinds of adrenal-stimulators—peanuts, salami, Roquefort cheese, and other salty, savory foods— throughout the "cocktail hour." A-types are also inclined to drink then; with their great energy, they seem to be particularly attracted to the relaxation of alcohol. Both habits can add vast numbers of calories to your daily total.

YOUR BEST SNACK IS
NO SNACK AT ALL

The fact that your adrenals are actually increasing in activity as the day progresses means that you should not, technically, have to snack at all. All you really have to do is wait and drink mineral water or Parsley Tea, or have a serving of your A-Type Vegetable Soup.

If you must snack, the best thing to do is to take half a carton of yogurt or half a glass of skim milk. By giving this stimulation to your pituitary and skipping a salty snack, you can also avoid another temptation for your body type, the desire to have an alcoholic drink.

THE A-TYPE HERBAL HELP: PARSLEY TEA

The herbal tea that does most for you is Parsley Tea. It has a refreshing, astringent quality that will satisfy your desire for a savory taste; this is in addition to its purifying effect on the adrenal glands.

It is paradoxical that you A-types, who are known for your hearty appetites, are very good dieters once you get started. The reason is the basic strength of the adrenal-type metabolism. It is quite rare for you to be overwhelmed by cravings, because your adrenals give you so much energy. But, of course, no one is completely immune from cravings, so if it should happen that you do get a strong desire to eat something salty and fattening, a cup of parsley tea will get you over it in no time.

Parsley Tea is made by adding a teaspoon of dried (not fresh) parsley leaves for each cup of tea you want to boiling water. Allow to steep for five minutes but do not boil the leaves. Strain and serve. You may add a half teaspoon of sugar or honey to this tea if you wish.

RULES FOR A-TYPE DIETING

In the following pages are both general guidelines for A-types (a complete list of exactly what you are to eat for each meal, for the Basic A-Type Weight Loss Diet and the A-Type Last Five Pounds Diet), and a week of sample menus for each of the diets. You may use these menus or substitute you own, as long as you use only the permitted foods and follow the guidelines given.

You may substitute within the boundaries allowed for each meal, but may not rearrange the food among the meals. Meat may only be boiled, grilled or barbecued or baked, with all visible fat removed (see the guidelines for each meal). Vegetables may be steamed, broiled with a small amount of oil, or sauteed in the permitted vegetable oil only. Poultry is to be eaten without skin. *Do not omit anything; every food is there for a reason.*

THE COMPLETE ADRENAL-TYPE WEIGHT LOSS PROGRAM

Your program begins with the Basic A-Type Weight Loss Diet. What happens after that depends on how much weight you want and need to lose.

TO LOSE MORE THAN FIFTEEN POUNDS: Follow the Basic A-Type Weight Loss Diet for three weeks, then change to the A-Type Last Five Pounds Diet for a week. Then go back to the Basic A-Type Weight Loss Diet, continuing to change to the Last Five Pounds Diet every fourth week. Once you are within five pounds of your ideal weight, use the Last Five Pounds Diet to lose these last stubborn pounds.

TO LOSE FIVE TO FIFTEEN POUNDS: Follow the Basic A-Type Weight Loss Diet for two weeks, then change to the A-Type Last Five Pounds Diet for a week (or less, if you reach your ideal weight before the week is done).

TO LOSE FIVE POUNDS OR LESS: Follow the Basic A-Type Weight Loss Diet for one week and go to the A-Type Last Five Pounds Diet for a week (or less).

WHEN YOU REACH YOUR IDEAL WEIGHT: Change to the A-Type Health and Weight Maintenance Diet.

Dishes which are marked with an asterisk are those for which a recipe is provided in Appendix 2.

THE BASIC A-TYPE WEIGHT LOSS DIET: GENERAL GUIDELINES

BREAKFAST

Choose either: 1 cup of yogurt OR 1 cup of lowfat cottage cheese OR 1 cup of whole-grain cereal with ½ cup of skim milk

Coffee, tea or Parsley Tea (½ teaspoon of sugar permitted)

WAIT FOUR HOURS

LUNCH

Large green salad made with any combination of lettuce, cucumber, mushrooms, celery, sprouts, radishes, bell pepper, tomato or onion

1 teaspoon of any clear diet dressing

Choice of ½ cup of beets, carrots, cauliflower, peas, pumpkin, squash or turnip

Choice of 1 cup of yogurt OR 1 cup of lowfat cottage cheese OR 4 ounces of lowfat hard cheese (such as Parmesan) OR 4 ounces of fish (but not shellfish)

Choice of 1 apple or: 2 apricots, ½ banana, 1 cup of berries, ¼ cantaloupe, 10 cherries, 2 figs, ½ mango, 1 nectarine, 1 peach, 1 pear, ½ cup of pineapple, 2 plums, 1 cup of watermelon or 1 cup of strawberries

Coffee, tea or Parsley Tea

WAIT SIX HOURS

DINNER

Choice of 4 ounces of chicken, 4 ounces of turkey, 4 ounces of fish, or 2 eggs

As much as you wish of zucchini, green pepper, snow peas, spinach, tomatoes or celery

2 teaspoons of vegetable oil (may be used in preparation of the poultry, fish or eggs, or on the vegetables)

1 cup of skim milk

Choice of the same fruits as for lunch OR 2 Chocolate Cookies* or Fruit Ice*

Parsley Tea

THE BASIC A-TYPE WEIGHT LOSS DIET: A WEEK OF SAMPLE MENUS

MONDAY

BREAKFAST: 1 cup of plain yogurt
Coffee or tea (with 1 teaspoon of sugar if desired)

LUNCH: Large green salad with clear diet dressing*
4 ounces of broiled fresh salmon, or 4 ounces water-packed canned salmon (salt rinsed out)
1 piece of rye Krispbread
1 peach
Coffee, tea or Parsley Tea (with 1 teaspoon of sugar if desired)

DINNER: Stir-fried Flank Steak* (or substitute your own recipe, using only 4 ounces of meat and any vegetables)
½ cup of white rice
1 piece of fruit
1 glass of skim milk
Parsley Tea (with 1 teaspoon of sugar if desired)

TUESDAY

BREAKFAST: 1 cup of lowfat cottage cheese
Coffee or tea (with 1 teaspoon of sugar if desired)

LUNCH: Large green salad with clear diet dressing*
                1 cup of plain yogurt with 1 cup of sliced straw-
                    berries
                1 slice of whole-wheat bread
                Coffee, Tea or Parsley Tea (with 1 teaspoon of
                    sugar if desired)

DINNER: Red Snapper "Scallops"* (or use your own fish
                    recipe, as long as the fish isn't breaded and
                    you use the permitted oil only)
                Steamed fresh spinach
                1 slice of french bread
                ½ cup of Fruit Ice*
                1 glass of skim milk
                Parsley Tea (with 1 teaspoon of sugar if desired)

WEDNESDAY

BREAKFAST: 1 cup of whole-grain cereal with ½ cup of skim
                    milk
                Coffee or tea (with 1 teaspoon of sugar if de-
                    sired)

LUNCH: Large green salad with clear diet dressing*
                4 ounces of water-packed tuna with celery and 1
                    teaspoon of diet mayonnaise
                1 slice of whole-grain bread
                1 bunch of grapes (about a cup)
                Coffee, tea or Parsley Tea (with 1 teaspoon of
                    sugar if desired)

DINNER: Chicken Burgers* (or your own chicken recipe,
                    as long as you use the permitted oil only, and
                    remove the skin)
                Steamed zucchini and string beans
                ½ cup of bulghur wheat*
                1 glass of skim milk
                1 piece of fruit
                Parsley Tea (with 1 teaspoon of sugar if desired)

THURSDAY

BREAKFAST: 1 cup of plain yogurt
Coffee or tea (with 1 teaspoon of sugar if desired)

LUNCH: Large green salad with clear diet dressing*
4 ounces of poached fish (or use your own fish recipe, preparing the fish without breading or added oil)
1 small baked or boiled potato
1 apple
Coffee, tea or Parsley Tea (with 1 teaspoon of sugar if desired)

DINNER: Turkey Kabobs* (or substitute your own turkey recipe, and do not eat the skin)
Cole slaw made with cabbage and 2 teaspoons of diet mayonnaise only
1 glass of skim milk
1 piece of rye Krispbread
2 Chocolate Cookies*
Parsley Tea (with 1 teaspoon of sugar if desired)

FRIDAY

BREAKFAST: 1 cup of lowfat cottage cheese
Coffee or tea (with 1 teaspoon of sugar if desired)

LUNCH: Large green salad with clear diet dressing*
4 ounces of Parmesan cheese toasted on
1 slice of whole-grain bread
1 cup of fresh cherries
Iced tea or Parsley Tea (with 1 teaspoon of sugar if desired)

DINNER: 1½ cups Chicken Vegetable Soup* (or use your own chicken recipe, using only permitted oil and omitting the skin)

1 small matzoh ball or dumpling
1 piece of fruit
1 glass of skim milk
Parsley Tea (with 1 teaspoon of sugar if desired)

SATURDAY

BREAKFAST: 1 cup of hot whole-grain cereal with ½ cup of skim milk
Coffee or tea (with 1 teaspoon of sugar if desired)

LUNCH: Large green salad with clear diet dressing*
4 ounces of water-packed tuna
1 slice of French bread
½ cantaloupe
Coffee, tea or Parsley Tea (with 1 teaspoon of sugar if desired)

DINNER: 4 ounces broiled steak (or you may substitute poultry or fish)
½ cup of bulghur wheat*
Steamed zucchini
1 glass of skim milk
1 piece of fruit
Parsley Tea (with 1 teaspoon of sugar if desired)

SUNDAY

BREAKFAST: 1 bowl of whole-grain cereal with ½ cup of skim milk
Coffee or tea (with 1 teaspoon of sugar if desired)

LUNCH: Large green salad with clear diet dressing*
4 ounces of Ceviche with Melon* (or substitute your own fish recipe according to A-Type guidelines)
2 sesame crackers

Coffee, tea or Parsley Tea (with 1 teaspoon of sugar if desired)

DINNER: Eggs Mornay* (you may substitute your own egg recipe or make a 2-egg omelette)
Spinach and mushroom salad
½ cup of Fruit Ice*
1 glass of skim milk
Parsley Tea (with 1 teaspoon of sugar if desired)

THE A-TYPE LAST FIVE POUNDS DIET

Remember, even if you have only five pounds of extra weight to lose, you should not begin the A-Type Last Five Pounds Diet until you have followed the Basic A-Type Weight Loss Diet for a week. The sequence of diets is vital, not only for losing weight but in bringing about a balance in your metabolism.

The A-Type Last Five Pounds Diet is a very special diet. It is a rapid weight-loss diet, containing only about 900 calories per day, 300 calories less than the Basic Weight Loss Diet. If you were to begin this diet immediately at the start of your dieting program, you would probably feel quite hungry on it. However, since you have followed the A-Type Basic Weight Loss Diet for at least a week, your metabolism has been strengthened and your balance improved. This means that you will not feel as hungry on your Last Five Pounds Diet as you otherwise would.

This diet is only to be followed for a week at a time. If at the end of a week you are not at your ideal weight, change back to the Basic A-Type Weight Loss Diet for one, two or three weeks, depending on your remaining extra weight. You change to the A-Type Last Five Pounds Diet every fourth week, or whenever you are within five pounds of your ideal weight. Once you have reached your ideal weight, you are ready for the A-Type Health and Weight Maintenance Program (see Chapter 10 for the complete program).

The days you spend on the Last Five Pounds Diet are the most important of your dieting career. These are the days when your body is most active in burning fat and in ridding itself of cellulite, the wrinkly fat which is the most difficult of all to lose. The loss of cellulite you will experience at this time indicates that your body is reaching a positive state of balance among the glands. Without this equilibrium, you always have the potential for becoming overweight again; but once you have it, you will be able to maintain your ideal weight with ease.

Note that the interval between meals is longer than on the Basic Weight Loss Diet. Be sure to observe these intervals; they are a vital part of your success.

THE A-TYPE LAST FIVE POUNDS DIET: GENERAL GUIDELINES

BREAKFAST

1 cup of plain yogurt OR 1 cup of lowfat cottage cheese OR 1 cup of whole-grain cereal with ½ cup skim milk

Coffee, tea or Parsley Tea (1 teaspoon of sugar allowed, if you wish)

WAIT FIVE HOURS

LUNCH

A-Type Vegetable Soup,* as much as you like

1 slice of whole-grain bread (without butter)

1 piece of fruit (choice of 1 apple, 2 apricots, ½ banana, 1 cup of berries, ¼ cantaloupe, 10 cherries, 2 fresh figs, ½ mango, 1 nectarine, 1 peach, 1 pear, ½ cup of fresh pineapple, 2 plums, 1 cup of strawberries or 1 cup of watermelon)

Parsley Tea (with 1 teaspoon of sugar allowed, if you wish)

WAIT SIX HOURS

DINNER

4 ounces of chicken OR 4 ounces of turkey OR 4 ounces of fish (not shellfish) OR 2 eggs

1 teaspoon of vegetable oil or butter

½ cup of brown rice OR ½ cup of bulghur wheat OR ½ cup of millet* OR 1 slice of whole-grain bread

A-Type Vegetable Soup,* as much as you like

Parsley Tea

A-TYPE LAST FIVE POUNDS DIET: A WEEK OF SAMPLE MENUS

MONDAY

BREAKFAST:
1 cup of plain yogurt
Coffee, tea or Parsley Tea (1 teaspoon of sugar if desired)

LUNCH:
A-Type Vegetable Soup* (as much as you like)
1 slice of whole-grain bread
1 piece of fruit, your choice
Coffee, tea or Parsley Tea (with 1 teaspoon of sugar if desired)

DINNER:
Chicken Breast Piquant*
½ cup of rice
A-Type Vegetable Soup*
Parsley Tea (with 1 teaspoon of sugar if desired)

TUESDAY

BREAKFAST:
1 cup of lowfat cottage cheese
Coffee, tea or Parsley Tea (1 teaspoon of sugar if desired)

LUNCH:
A-Type Vegetable Soup* (as much as you like)
1 slice of whole-grain bread
1 piece of fruit, your choice
Coffee, tea or Parsley Tea (with 1 teaspoon of sugar if desired)

DINNER:
Turkey Kabobs*
½ cup of bulghur wheat*
A-Type Vegetable Soup*
Parsley Tea (with 1 teaspoon of sugar if desired)

WEDNESDAY

BREAKFAST: 1 cup of whole-grain cereal with ½ cup of skim milk
Coffee, tea or Parsley Tea (1 teaspoon of sugar if desired)

LUNCH: A-Type Vegetable Soup* (as much as you like)
1 slice of whole-grain bread
1 piece of fruit, your choice
Coffee, tea or Parsley Tea (with 1 teaspoon of sugar if desired)

DINNER: Fish Veronique A-Type*
½ cup of millet*
A-Type Vegetable Soup*
Parsley Tea (with 1 teaspoon of sugar if desired)

THURSDAY

BREAKFAST: 1 cup of plain yogurt
Coffee, tea or Parsley Tea (1 teaspoon of sugar if desired)

LUNCH: A-Type Vegetable Soup* (as much as you like)
1 slice of whole-grain bread
1 piece of fruit, your choice
Coffee, tea or Parsley Tea (with 1 teaspoon of sugar if desired)

DINNER: Chicken Burgers*
½ whole-wheat burger bun
A-Type Vegetable Soup
Parsley Tea (with 1 teaspoon of sugar if desired)

FRIDAY

BREAKFAST: 1 cup of lowfat cottage cheese
Coffee, tea or Parsley Tea (1 teaspoon of sugar if desired)

LUNCH: A-Type Vegetable Soup* (as much as you like)
1 slice of whole-grain bread
1 piece of fruit, your choice
Coffee, tea or Parsley Tea (with 1 teaspoon of sugar if desired)

DINNER: Herb Omelette*
½ cup of rice
A-Type Vegetable Soup*
Parsley Tea (with 1 teaspoon of sugar if desired)

SATURDAY

BREAKFAST: 1 cup of whole-grain cereal with ½ cup of skim milk
Coffee, tea or Parsley Tea (1 teaspoon of sugar if desired)

LUNCH: A-Type Vegetable Soup* (as much as you like)
1 slice of whole-grain bread
1 piece of fruit, your choice
Coffee, tea or Parsley Tea (with 1 teaspoon of sugar if desired)

DINNER: Sole Provencal*
½ cup of bulghur wheat*
A-Type Vegetable Soup*
Parsley Tea (with 1 teaspoon of sugar if desired)

SUNDAY

BREAKFAST: 1 cup of plain yogurt
Coffee, tea or Parsley Tea (1 teaspoon of sugar if desired)

LUNCH: A-Type Vegetable Soup* (as much as you like)
1 slice of whole-grain bread
1 piece of fruit, your choice
Coffee, tea or Parsley Tea (with 1 teaspoon of sugar if desired)

R: Lemon Chicken Kabobs*
½ cup of millet*
A-Type Vegetable Soup*
Parsley Tea (with 1 teaspoon of sugar if desired)

THE A-TYPE HEALTH AND WEIGHT MAINTENANCE PROGRAM

The formula for keeping the ideal weight you've achieved through your Body Type Diet is to have a continuing awareness of your body type and its special needs. Your A-Type Weight Loss Program has brought about a state of balance in your metabolism; the A-Type Health and Weight Maintenance Program is designed to make it easy for you to *maintain* that balance, and to keep your ideal weight.

"PLENTY," "MODERATION" AND "RARELY" FOODS

To make it as easy as possible for you to keep your body type requirements in mind, your program includes a *short, simple* set of guidelines for your body type. You need only remember: 1) your Plenty Foods (foods you can always eat, which will always be good for you); 2) your Moderation Foods (foods you can eat as long as you don't overdo them—I'll indicate your safe quantity of them), and 3) your Rarely Foods (ones you should save for special occasions only, because eating them will tend to revive your old cravings and make it harder for you to keep to your guidelines).

Continue to use your Herbal Tea and your Vegetable Soup. They will continue to strengthen your metabolism and are the best possible means for you to maintain the healthy balance you have achieved.

IF YOU FORGET THE GUIDELINES AND GAIN WEIGHT

If you stay with your guidelines you will not find yourself putting on weight. But if you let your guidelines go for a while (for instance, during a holiday season or on a vacation) and you find yourself three to five pounds above your ideal weight, then go back to the A-Type Weight Loss Program. With five extra pounds, you will need only a week of your A-Type Weight Loss Diet and a weekend of the A-Type Last Five Pounds Diet to be right back at your perfect weight.

THE A-TYPE HEALTH AND WEIGHT MAINTENANCE PROGRAM: GENERAL GUIDELINES

1. YOUR PLENTY FOODS:
   Yogurt
   Cottage cheese
   Diet American cheese
   String cheese
   Skim milk
   Fruit
   Fresh vegetables
   Whole grains
   Parsley Tea

2. YOUR MODERATION FOODS:
   Fish
   Poultry
   Coffee or tea
   Light desserts
   Vegetable oils

3. YOUR RARELY FOODS:
   Salty foods
   Yellow or Aged Cheese
   Red meat
   Butter
   Shellfish

4. YOUR IDEAL EATING SCHEDULE:
   A light breakfast of dairy products or whole grains

   A fairly light lunch, with only a small amount of protein

   Your main meal at night

BREAKFAST

A serving of yogurt OR cottage cheese OR a bowl of whole-grain cereal with skim milk

Coffee, tea or Parsley Tea (with one teaspoon of sugar if desired)

LUNCH

A large green salad with all your favorite vegetables, and clear diet dressing in moderation

A small serving of chicken or fish. Lamb or shellfish may be substituted once a week if you like

2 slices of whole-grain bread, or an equivalent serving of other whole grain

A glass of skim milk

A piece of fruit

Coffee, tea or Parsley Tea (with one teaspoon of sugar if desired)

DINNER

A serving of meat, fish or poultry. Eat meat 1 or 2 times a week only, poultry or fish the remaining days. Or, have 2 or more meatless dinners per week, using whole grains, eggs, nuts or dairy products

Vegetables, cooked or raw, as much as you like

A serving of grain, which should be whole grain 4 times a week at least

A piece of fruit or 2 Chocolate Cookies* or Fruit Ice*

Coffee, tea or Parsley Tea (with one teaspoon of sugar if desired)

8
THE THYROID BODY TYPE WEIGHT LOSS PROGRAM

THE BASIC STRATEGY FOR T-TYPES

The first and most important dieting strategy for you as a thyroid type is to reverse your habit of overstimulating your thyroid gland. As long as your thyroid is in its present, overstimulated state, you will *never* lose weight and keep it off.

You do this, first, but cutting out all refined carbohydrates (white flour, sugar, white rice, pasta and anything made with these ingredients). You cannot eliminate carbohydrates completely, for carbohydrates are an essential part of a healthy diet. But those you eat should be whole grains: brown rice, whole wheat, rye, or millet. In this way you supply your body with the carbohydrates you need, while avoiding the overstimulation of *refined* carbohydrate products.

NO FRUIT FOR NOW

You also do not eat fruit while dieting. Fruit is a "natural" food, unlike refined sugar and flour, but it contains too much thyroid-stimulating simple sugar for you while you are resting your thyroid. Later, when you have lost your excess weight and restored your metabolic balance, you can put back into your diet a moderate amount of fruit (three or four pieces per week). But you never can go back to eating sugary sweets; for you they are truly a drug, not a food.

ELIMINATE CAFFEINE

The elimination of caffeine for the duration of your weight loss period is also very important. This means no coffee, tea or cola—not even diet cola. Surprisingly, many soft drinks besides cola contain caffeine. Diet Mr. Pibbs and Diet Dr. Pepper are two sugar-free drinks which are very high in caffeine (see *Consumer Reports,* October 1981). I do not like diet soft drinks in general, but if you must drink them, Diet 7-Up and Diet Sunkist Orange at least have the advantage of being caffeine-free. Or drink carbonated mineral water or club soda instead. These drinks are refreshing, have no calories, and are so much kinder to the thyroid gland.

A cup of decaffeinated coffee or tea is permitted with your breakfast. Do without it if you can. Even "decaffeinated" drinks contain *some* caffeine. If you have been drinking a great deal of caffeine for years, you may find that cutting it out suddenly gives you a headache. Caffeine is mildly addictive and the headache is a withdrawal symptom. If this happens, cut down gradually on your consumption, reducing by a cup a day, until you are off caffeine entirely.

EAT EGGS EVERY DAY

The second aspect of your strategy is to build up your adrenals. The best way for you to do this is by eating eggs every day. Eggs supply a highly useful form of cholesterol which is used in the manufacture of adrenal hormones.

Start every day with two eggs for breakfast. My T-type patients sometimes protest that they can't look at anything but coffee and toast in the morning. But the eggs are a vital part of your strategy, and after a week or two on eggs for breakfast I see the most striking transformations of my patients. The stimulation of the adrenals does absolute wonders.

T-type men may be concerned about their cholesterol levels if they eat eggs every day. This is a controversial question on which all the evidence is not yet in, but the latest findings indicate that cholesterol in the diet has very little effect on *blood* cholesterol levels. However, you should consult your physician and follow his advice. If you are advised to restrict your egg intake, then substitute four ounces of white poultry meat for each two-egg serving in your diet. But if you *can* eat the eggs, you *should* eat the eggs.

EAT PLENTY OF POULTRY AND FISH, SOME RED MEAT, LOTS OF VEGETABLES

Besides eggs, the best adrenal-strengthening foods for you are chicken and other poultry, and fish. These light animal proteins are nourishing to your adrenals, but do not stimulate them too much, as eating a great deal of red meat would do. If you eat small portions of red meat two or three times a week, that is plenty.

You eat an abundance of vegetables, both raw in salads and lightly cooked. The vegetables supply vitamins, minerals and a feeling of fullness, so that you never feel deprived or "empty."

THE TOTAL STRATEGY

Your total dieting strategy, in summary, is: eggs every day, lots of protein from chicken and fish, a moderate amount of red meat, a small amount of carbohydrates from whole-grain sources, lots of fresh vegetables and salads, and no fruit.

As a result, you'll have steadier energy throughout the day. You'll be less nervous and irritable. Your fat will come off more quickly than you've ever imagined it could, and you'll enjoy a dramatic loss of your cellulite, especially during the Last Five Pounds phase of your diet.

THE T-TYPE MEAL SCHEDULE

EAT THREE EQUAL MEALS A DAY

The most important factor in T-type timing is the necessity to steady your energy and reduce its up-and-down quality. This is done by distributing your caloric intake evenly among the three meals.

You may have been in the habit of skipping breakfast, or having only coffee and toast or a pastry, but this is a mistake. If you eat a thyroid-stimulating breakfast like this you'll be nervous and hungry by midmorning, will "need" another cup of coffee, a cola, or a sweet, and will be eating thyroid-stimulating foods all day.

OBSERVE THE INTERVALS BETWEEN MEALS

You must be careful to observe the intervals I specify between meals. These are four hours between breakfast and lunch and six hours between lunch and dinner on the Basic T-Type Weight Loss Diet, and *five* hours between breakfast and lunch and six hours between lunch and dinner on the Last Five Pounds Diet. These are the intervals in which fat is burned. If you start eating too soon after eating the last meal, you will not get the full benefit of your Body Type Diet.

YOUR DANGER PERIODS

The danger period for T-type cravings is whenever the thyroid gland is low. Unfortunately, this can happen at any time. The key to knowing when it will be low is to realize that it will happen at definite intervals following stimulation of the gland with starches or caffeine.

Thyroid fatigue occurs in two waves. First there is a wave of tiredness (accompanied by the urge to snack) about an hour and a half after stimulation; then there is a second wave of fatigue three to four hours later.

YOUR BEST SNACK

Even though eating eggs for breakfast, and eliminating caffeine, does a great deal to mitigate thyroidal fatigue, you may still find you have an urge to snack in the late afternoon, when the thyroid is naturally least active. This is the time to have, not a thyroid-stimulator, but half a hard-boiled egg. I tell my T-type patients always to keep a hard-boiled egg or two in the refrigerator, so it's easier to have one than to take a cookie. Do this. It works. One of the most exhausted T-types I ever met was a young woman who ate half a cookie whenever she wanted because "it didn't count."

THE T-TYPE HERBAL HELP: RASPBERRY LEAF TEA

Raspberry Leaf Tea will help you immeasurably on your Weight Loss Program. Drink as much of it as you like, but be sure to drink at least the amounts called for in your diet. If you have a cup at moments when you are experiencing cravings, you will find that your craving often vanishes, since the tea both soothes and strengthens your metabolism.

Make Raspberry Leaf Tea like this: Bring water to a boil. Add the boiling water to a teaspoon of raspberry leaves for each cup of water. Allow to steep for five minutes, strain and serve. Don't add any sugar or honey—they're thyroid-stimulators. In any case, the taste is pleasant. Raspberry leaves are available in most health food stores.

RULES FOR T-TYPE DIETING

In the following pages are both general guidelines for T-type dieting (a complete list of exactly what you can eat for each meal, both for the Basic Weight Loss Diet and the Last Five Pounds Diet) and a week of sample menus for each of the diets. You may use the sample menus or substitute your own, as long as you use only the permitted foods and follow the guidelines exactly.

You may substitute only within the boundaries allowed for each meal, but may not rearrange the food among meals. Meat may only be broiled, grilled, or baked (see guidelines for each meal). Vegetables may be steamed, boiled in a small amount of water, or sauteed in the permitted vegetable oil only. Poultry is to be eaten without skin. *Do not omit anything; every food is there for a reason.*

THE COMPLETE
THYROID-TYPE
WEIGHT LOSS
PROGRAM

Your program begins with one week of the Basic T-Type Weight Loss Diet. How long you follow it depends on how much weight you want to lose.

TO LOSE MORE THAN FIFTEEN POUNDS: Follow the Basic T-Type Weight Loss Diet for three weeks, then change to the T-Type Last Five Pounds Diet for a week. Then go back to the Basic T-Type Weight Loss Diet, changing to the T-Type Last Five Pounds Diet every fourth week for as long as needed. Once you are within five pounds of your ideal weight, use the Last Five Pounds Diet and finish your weight loss program with it.

TO LOSE FIVE TO FIFTEEN POUNDS: Follow the Basic T-Type Weight Loss Diet for two weeks, then the T-Type Last Five Pounds Diet for a week (or less, if you reach your ideal weight before the end of the week).

TO LOSE FIVE POUNDS OR LESS: Follow the Basic T-Type Weight Loss Diet for one week and then the T-Type Last Five Pounds Diet for a week (or less).

WHEN YOU REACH YOUR IDEAL WEIGHT: Begin the T-Type Health and Weight Maintenance Program.

Dishes marked with an asterisk are those for which a recipe is provided in Appendix 3.

THE BASIC T-TYPE WEIGHT LOSS DIET: GENERAL GUIDELINES

BREAKFAST

2 eggs, any style

1 teaspoon of butter or oil (use either to cook the eggs, or on the toast)

½ slice of whole-grain bread or toast

1 cup only of decaffeinated coffee or tea, or Raspberry Leaf Tea

WAIT FOUR HOURS

LUNCH

Large green salad of any combination of lettuce, cucumber, mushrooms, celery, sprouts, radishes, bell pepper, tomato and onion

1 teaspoon of any clear diet dressing (not creamy or spicy)

1 teaspoon of butter or diet mayonnaise

Choice of either: 4 ounces of poultry OR 4 ounces of fish

Choice of either: 1 slice of whole-grain bread OR ½ cup of bulghur wheat OR ½ cup of brown rice OR ½ cup of millet*

1 cup of skim milk

Raspberry Leaf Tea

WAIT SIX HOURS

DINNER

Choice of 4 ounces of chicken OR 4 ounces of turkey OR 4 ounces of fish OR 4 ounces of lamb with fat cut off OR 4 ounces of organ meat (liver, kidneys or heart)* OR 4 ounces of lean beef. (NOTE: have beef 2 or 3 times a week only)

Raw or steamed vegetables, your choice, as much as you wish

Choice of 1 slice of whole-grain bread OR ½ cup of bulghur wheat OR ½ cup of brown rice OR ½ cup of millet*—no butter

1 cup of skim milk

Raspberry Leaf Tea

THE BASIC T-TYPE WEIGHT LOSS DIET: A WEEK OF SAMPLE MENUS

MONDAY

BREAKFAST: 2 scrambled eggs cooked in 1 teaspoon of vegetable oil
½ slice of whole-wheat toast
Decaffeinated coffee, 1 cup only

LUNCH: Large green salad with clear diet dressing*
4 ounces of water-packed tuna
1 teaspoon of diet mayonnaise
1 glass of skim milk
Raspberry Leaf Tea

DINNER: Mexican Stuffed Chicken* (or use your own chicken recipe, preparing the chicken with skin and with 1 teaspoon of vegetable oil only)
½ cup of brown rice*
Cucumber salad dressed with 1 tablespoon of yogurt
1 glass of skim milk
Raspberry Leaf Tea

TUESDAY

BREAKFAST: 2 poached eggs
½ slice of whole-grain toast
1 teaspoon of butter
Decaffeinated tea, 1 cup only

LUNCH: Large green salad with clear diet dressing
4 ounces of cooked chicken
1 teaspoon of butter or mayonnaise

½ of a whole-grain English muffin
1 glass of skim milk
Raspberry Leaf Tea

DINNER: Baked Halibut Steak* (or use your own fish rec-
               ipe, prepared without breading or added oil)
               Steamed spinach, as much as you like
               ½ cup of millet*
               1 glass of skim milk
               Raspberry Leaf Tea

WEDNESDAY

BREAKFAST: 2 fried eggs, cooked in 1 teaspoon of vegetable
               oil
               ½ slice of seven-grain toast
               Raspberry Leaf Tea

LUNCH: 4 ounces of canned salmon (fresh if available)
               1 slice of whole-grain bread
               1 teaspoon of butter or diet mayonnaise
               Large green salad with clear diet dressing*
               1 glass of skim milk
               Raspberry Leaf Tea

DINNER: 4 ounces of lean steak, broiled
               Steamed zucchini and string beans
               1 teaspoon of butter on the vegetables
               1 small baked potato
               1 glass of skim milk
               Raspberry Leaf Tea

THURSDAY

BREAKFAST: 2 eggs, scrambled, cooked in 1 teaspoon of vege-
               table oil
               ½ slice of whole wheat toast
               Decaffeinated coffee, 1 cup only

LUNCH: 4 ounces of sliced turkey
1 teaspoon of diet mayonnaise
Large green salad with clear diet dressing*
2 pieces of rye Krispbread
1 glass of skim milk
Raspberry Leaf Tea

DINNER: Barbecued Tuna* (or use your own fish recipe,
using no breading and 1 teaspoon of vegetable
oil only)
Steamed carrots with parsley
½ cup of bulghur wheat*
1 glass of skim milk
Raspberry Leaf Tea

FRIDAY

BREAKFAST: 2 hard-boiled eggs
½ slice of rye toast with 1 teaspoon of butter
Decaffeinated tea, 1 cup only

LUNCH: 4 ounces of water-packed tuna
1 teaspoon of diet mayonnaise
Large green salad with clear diet dressing*
1 glass of skim milk
1 slice of rye toast
Raspberry Leaf Tea

DINNER: Chicken Stew* (or use your own chicken recipe,
prepared without skin or added oil)
1 whole-wheat roll
1 glass of skim milk
Raspberry Leaf Tea

SATURDAY

BREAKFAST: 2 poached eggs
½ whole-grain English muffin, 1 teaspoon of butter
Decaffeinated coffee, 1 cup only

LUNCH: Chef's Salad*
           2 pieces of rye Krispbread
           Large green salad with clear diet dressing*
           1 glass of skim milk
           Raspberry Leaf Tea

DINNER: Sesame Shrimp with Asparagus* (or use your
           own shrimp recipe, using no breading and 1
           teaspoon of vegetable oil only)
           ½ cup of brown rice*
           Steamed green beans, as much as you like
           1 glass of skim milk
           Raspberry Leaf Tea

SUNDAY

BREAKFAST: Omelette with Herbs*
           ½ slice of whole-grain bread
           Decaffeinated coffee, 1 cup only

LUNCH: 4 ounces of broiled chicken breast
           1 slice of rye toast
           Large green salad with clear diet dressing*
           1 glass of skim milk
           Raspberry Leaf Tea

DINNER: 4 ounces of roast lamb
           1 teaspoon of mint sauce (not mint jelly)
           1 small baked potato
           1 teaspoon of butter
           1 glass of skim milk
           Raspberry Leaf Tea

THE T-TYPE LAST FIVE POUNDS DIET

Remember, even if you have only five pounds of extra weight, you should not begin your T-Type Last Five Pounds Diet until you have followed the Basic T-Type Weight Loss Diet for a week. The sequence of diets is vital for balancing your metabolism, as well as for producing fast efficient loss of weight.

The T-Type Last Five Pounds Diet is a very special diet. It has just over 900 calories per day, about 300 calories per day less than the Basic T-Type Weight Loss Diet; and the food you eat is specially programmed to get you off the periodic plateaus of dieting, as well as to assist you in losing the stubborn last five pounds of excess weight. If you were to begin this diet at the start of your program you would probably find it difficult. But since you have been on the Basic T-Type Weight Loss Diet for at least a week, your metabolism is strengthened and in better balance, and you will be able to handle the Last Five Pounds Diet comfortably.

This diet is only to be followed for a week at a time. If, at the end of a week, you have not reached your ideal weight, return to the Basic T-Type Weight Loss Diet for one, two or three weeks, depending on your situation; you may use the Last Five Pounds Diet every fourth week until you reach your weight goal. And as soon as you come within five pounds of your ideal weight, change to the Last Five Pounds Diet to lose that last bit of weight.

Note that the interval of time between meals has been increased on the Last Five Pounds Diet. Be sure to observe the full interval, as the hours between meals are the periods when your body is most active in burning fat.

THE T-TYPE LAST FIVE POUNDS DIET: GENERAL GUIDELINES

BREAKFAST

2 eggs, any style

1 teaspoon of vegetable oil

T-Type Vegetable Soup,* as much as you like

Raspberry Leaf Tea

WAIT FIVE HOURS

LUNCH

4 ounces of fish or shellfish

T-Type Vegetable Soup,* as much as you like

Raspberry Leaf Tea

WAIT SIX HOURS

DINNER

Choice of: 4 ounces of poultry OR 4 ounces of fish OR 4 ounces of shellfish

T-Type Vegetable Soup,* as much as you like

Choice of: ½ cup of millet OR ½ cup of brown rice OR ½ cup of bulghur wheat* OR 1 slice of whole-grain bread

Raspberry Leaf Tea

THE T-TYPE LAST FIVE POUNDS DIET: A WEEK OF SAMPLE MENUS

MONDAY

BREAKFAST: Two eggs, any style, cooked in 1 teaspoon of vegetable oil
T-Type Vegetable Soup*
Raspberry Leaf Tea

LUNCH: T-Type Vegetable Soup* (as much as you like)
4 ounces of water-packed tuna
Raspberry Leaf Tea

DINNER: Chicken Piquant* (or use your own chicken recipe, preparing chicken without skin and with 1 teaspoon of vegetable oil)
T-Type Vegetable Soup* (as much as you like)
½ cup of brown rice*
Raspberry Leaf Tea

TUESDAY

BREAKFAST: 2 eggs, any style, cooked in 1 teaspoon of vegetable oil
T-Type Vegetable Soup*
Raspberry Leaf Tea

LUNCH: T-Type Vegetable Soup* (as much as you like)
4 ounces of fresh or canned salmon
Raspberry Leaf Tea

DINNER: Turkey Kabobs* (or use your own turkey recipe, preparing turkey without skin)
T-Type Vegetable Soup* (as much as you like)
1 slice of whole-grain bread
Raspberry Leaf Tea

WEDNESDAY

BREAKFAST: 2 eggs, any style, cooked in 1 teaspoon of vege-
table oil
T-Type Vegetable Soup*
Raspberry Leaf Tea

LUNCH: T-Type Vegetable Soup* (as much as you like)
4 ounces of Broiled Shrimp with Lemon*
Raspberry Leaf Tea

DINNER: Baked Halibut Steak* (or use your own fish recipe, prepared without breading and with 1 teaspoon of vegetable oil)
T-Type Vegetable Soup* (as much as you like)
½ cup of bulghur wheat*
Raspberry Leaf Tea

THURSDAY

BREAKFAST: 2 eggs, any style, cooked in 1 teaspoon of vege-
table oil
T-Type Vegetable Soup*
Raspberry Leaf Tea

LUNCH: T-Type Vegetable Soup* (as much as you like)
4 ounces of water-packed tuna
Raspberry Leaf Tea

DINNER: Stir-Fried Chicken* (or use your own chicken
recipe)
T-Type Vegetable Soup* (as much as you like)
½ cup of millet*
Raspberry Leaf Tea

FRIDAY

BREAKFAST: 2 eggs, any style, cooked in 1 teaspoon of vege-
table oil
T-Type Vegetable Soup*
Raspberry Leaf Tea

LUNCH: T-Type Vegetable Soup* (as much as you like)
            4 ounces of broiled scallops
            Raspberry Leaf Tea

DINNER: Herb Omelette* (or use your own egg recipe,
            using 2 eggs and 1 teaspoon of vegetable oil)
            T-Type Vegetable Soup* (as much as you like)
            ½ cup of brown rice*
            Raspberry Leaf Tea

SATURDAY

BREAKFAST: 2 eggs, any style, cooked in 1 teaspoon of vege-
            table oil
            T-Type Vegetable Soup*
            Raspberry Leaf Tea

LUNCH: T-Type Vegetable Soup* (as much as you like)
            4 ounces water-packed canned shrimp
            Raspberry Leaf Tea

DINNER: Chicken Stew* (or use your own chicken recipe,
            cooking chicken without skin)
            T-Type Vegetable Soup* (as much as you like)
            ½ cup of bulghur wheat*
            Raspberry Leaf Tea

SUNDAY

BREAKFAST: 2 eggs, any style, cooked in 1 teaspoon of vege-
            table oil
            T-Type Vegetable Soup*
            Raspberry Leaf Tea

LUNCH: T-Type Vegetable Soup* (as much as you like)
            4 ounces of fresh or canned salmon
            Raspberry Leaf Tea

DINNER: Salmon Steak Florentine* (or use your own fish
            recipe, using no breading and 1 teaspoon of
            vegetable oil only)

T-Type Vegetable Soup* (as much as you like)
½ cup of millet*
Raspberry Leaf Tea

THE T-TYPE HEALTH AND WEIGHT MAINTENANCE PROGRAM

The formula for keeping the ideal weight you've achieved through your Body Type Diet is to have a continuing awareness of your body type and its special needs. Your T-Type Diet has brought about a state of balance in your metabolism; the T-Type Health and Weight Maintenance Program is designed to make it easy for you to *maintain* that balance, and to keep your ideal weight.

"PLENTY," "MODERATION" AND "RARELY" FOODS

To make it as easy as possible for you to keep your body type requirements in mind, your program begins with a *short, simple* set of guidelines for your body type. You need only keep in mind: 1) your Plenty Foods (foods you can always eat, which will always be good for you); 2) your Moderation Foods (foods you can eat as long as you don't overdo them—I'll indicate your safe quantity of them); and 3) your Rarely Foods (ones you should save for special occasions only, because eating them will tend to revive your old cravings and make it harder for you to keep to your guidelines).

Continue to use your Herbal Tea and your Vegetable Soup. They will continue to strengthen your metabolism and are the best possible means for you to maintain the healthy balance you have achieved.

IF YOU FORGET THE GUIDELINES AND GAIN WEIGHT

If you stay with your guidelines you will not find yourself putting on weight. But if you should let your guidelines go for any reason and you find yourself three to five pounds above your ideal weight, then go back to your original T-Type Weight Loss Program. With five extra pounds, you will need only a week of your T-Type Weight Loss Diet and a weekend of the T-Type Last Five Pounds Diet to be right back at your perfect weight.

THE T-TYPE HEALTH AND WEIGHT MAINTENANCE PROGRAM: GENERAL GUIDELINES

1. YOUR PLENTY FOODS:

Eggs
Poultry: chicken, turkey, game hen
Fresh vegetables
Raspberry Leaf Tea

2. YOUR MODERATION FOODS:

Red meat
Organ meats: liver, kidneys, heart
Cheese
Yogurt
Whole grains
Fruit
Decaffeinated coffee and tea
Butter, vegetable oils

3. YOUR RARELY FOODS:

Refined grains
Coffee
Tea
Sugary desserts

4. YOUR IDEAL EATING SCHEDULE:

Eggs for breakfast (a good lifetime habit for T-Types)

Your total food intake divided more or less evenly among your meals

Protein at each meal

A protein snack (e.g. half a hard-boiled egg) in the late afternoon if you feel tired

BREAKFAST

2 eggs, any style

1 slice of whole-grain toast with butter

Decaffeinated coffee, tea or Raspberry Leaf Tea

LUNCH

A large green salad with plenty of your favorite vegetables, clear diet dressing* used in moderation

A serving of hard cheese, yogurt or cottage cheese, OR a serving of meat or fish

2 slices of whole-grain bread, or an equivalent serving of other whole grains*

A glass of milk

A piece of fruit

Decaffeinated coffee, tea or Raspberry Leaf Tea

DINNER

A serving of meat, poultry or fish. Plan to eat meat about twice a week, fish or poultry on the remaining nights

Vegetables, cooked or raw, as much as you like

A serving of whole grain*

A glass of milk (optional)

A piece of fruit or a small dessert (but not more than twice a week!)

Raspberry Leaf Tea

9

THE PITUITARY BODY TYPE WEIGHT LOSS PROGRAM

THE BASIC STRATEGY FOR P-TYPES

Stimulating your adrenals is the single most important factor for Pituitary types. It corrects two problems at once: it improves the digestion, which allows you to burn fat more efficiently, and it gives you a steadier strength throughout the day, so that you are less inclined to snack.

The most effective adrenal-stimulating food is meat, especially beef. Organ meats—liver, kidneys, heart—also work well. Poultry and fish have some adrenal-stimulating qualities, and can be used to vary the diet. Organ meats have an additional advantage of stimulating the sex glands, which are also underactive in pituitary types.

ELIMINATE DAIRY PRODUCTS

The P-type metabolism works best when you eat no dairy products at all. After you have lost all your excess weight you may have a very occasional yogurt, but no more than that. The more faithfully you stay away from dairy products, the better you are going to feel.

AVOID REFINED CARBOHYDRATES AND CAFFEINE (WHOLE GRAINS ARE OK)

Your carbohydrate intake is from whole grains. The P-type metabolism does not need thyroidal stimulation; for this reason you avoid refined carbohydrates, including all kinds of sugar and honey, and white flour. You may have two pieces of fruit per day. Caffeine is to be avoided as it gives you too much thyroid stimulation. You may drink decaffeinated coffee if you wish.

EAT PLENTY OF FRESH VEGETABLES

You eat a large green salad every day at lunch, and as many vegetables as you wish at dinner, either cooked or raw. Vegetables provide vitamins, minerals and a feeling of fullness while dieting.

THE TOTAL STRATEGY

To summarize your total dieting strategy: no dairy products; plenty of protein from animal sources—emphasizing beef and organ meats, with chicken and fish for variety; carbohydrates in moderation but from whole-grain sources only; fruit in moderation; no sugar or white flour; no caffeine; and plenty of fresh vegetables, both cooked and raw.

As a result, your digestion will improve. Your metabolism will become more active, so you'll lose weight quicker. You'll feel more in touch with your body, and learn only to eat when you are actually hungry, and to stop when you are full. You'll lose stubborn fat and even your cellulite, especially during the Last Five Pounds phase of your diet. And, interestingly, you'll find your sexuality blossoming in a very natural way.

THE P-TYPE MEAL SCHEDULE

REVERSE THE "USUAL" ORDER OF MEALS

The pituitary gland is active during the day, especially early in the day, and relatively inactive at night. This makes you a "morning person"; your ideal schedule is early to bed, early to rise, for you have your best energy early in the day.

To lose weight most effectively, P-types must reverse the usual order of meals. Instead of a light breakfast, moderate lunch and substantial dinner, you should eat a substantial breakfast, with meat, a moderate lunch, and a very light dinner.

EAT A SUBSTANTIAL BREAKFAST WITH MEAT

Eating meat at breakfast accomplishes several purposes. It starts your day with the adrenal stimulation you need. It pulls your energies down into your body (by stimulating the lower glands, rather than the pituitary), which will help you focus during the day. It stays with you longer than your usual yogurt breakfast, and will help you avoid snacking. Finally, it keeps you more in touch with your body, which will help you know when you actually are hungry and so to avoid eating from nervousness or tension. Lunch should also contain some protein, to help you eliminate snacking throughout the afternoon.

EAT LIGHTLY AT NIGHT

Because your metabolism is so inactive late in the day, going to bed with a heavy meal on your stomach is always to be avoided. You'll only suffer from indigestion and disturbed sleep.

OBSERVE THE INTERVAL BETWEEN MEALS

Wait four hours between breakfast and lunch and six hours between lunch and dinner on the Basic P-Type Weight Loss Diet, five hours between breakfast and lunch and six between lunch and dinner on the P-Type Last Five Pounds Diet. It is vital that you keep to these intervals, which enable your body to complete the digestive process and to have some time, free of digestion, to rebalance itself. Eating too soon after a previous meal distracts your body from this vital process of rebalancing, which is also when the work of burning fat takes place.

YOUR DANGER PERIOD

Your danger period for snacking is late afternoon, as your pituitary gland becomes less and less active. At this time many P-types experience a desire for pituitary stimulation—ice cream, yogurt, cheese—or occasionally for a thyroid-stimulator such as a sweet or starch. These must be avoided at all costs.

YOUR BEST SNACK

Keep available in your refrigerator a small amount of already-cooked meat—for example, a few ounces of cooked hamburger well drained of fat. If you are overcome with the desire to snack, take a few bites of the meat instead. It will stimulate your adrenals and you'll feel more energetic, and you'll avoid sabotaging your diet with a pituitary or thyroid-stimulating food.

THE P-TYPE HERBAL HELP: FENUGREEK TEA

Fenugreek Tea is an important feature of the pituitary-type diet. Drink as much of it as you wish, but be sure to drink *at least* the amounts specified in your diet. And drink it any time you have a strong craving for ice cream or other dairy foods.

It is made as follows: Bring water to a boil and add a teaspoon of fenugreek seeds (available in most health food stores) for each two cups of water. Allow the seeds to boil in the water for five minutes. Unlike most herbal teas, Fenugreek Tea must be boiled to release the full value of the seeds. Strain and serve. You may use as much lemon as you wish, but no honey or sugar.

RULES FOR P-TYPE DIETING

In the following pages are both general guidelines for P-type dieting (a complete list of what you are to eat for each meal, both for the Basic P-Type Weight Loss Diet and the P-Type Last Five Pounds Diet) and a week of sample menus for each of the diets. Use these samples menus or substitute your own, as long as you use only the permitted foods and follow the guidelines exactly.

You may substitute only within the boundaries allowed for each meal, but may not rearrange the food among the meals. Meat may only be boiled, grilled, or baked, with all visible fat removed (see guidelines for each meal). Vegetables may be steamed, boiled in a small amount of water, or sauteed in the permitted vegetable oil only. Poultry is to be eaten without skin. *Do not omit anything; every food is there for a reason.*

THE COMPLETE
PITUITARY-TYPE
WEIGHT LOSS
PROGRAM

Your program begins with the P-Type Weight Loss Diet. How long you follow it depends on how much weight you want to lose.

TO LOSE MORE THAN FIFTEEN POUNDS: Follow the Basic P-Type Weight Loss Diet for three weeks, then change to the P-Type Last Five Pounds Diet for a week, then go back to the Basic P-Type Weight Loss Diet. Continue to change to the Last Five Pounds Diet every fourth week. Once you are within five pounds of your ideal weight, use the Last Five Pounds Diet to complete your weight loss program.

TO LOSE FIVE TO FIFTEEN POUNDS: Follow the Basic P-Type Weight Loss Diet for two weeks, then change to the P-Type Last Five Pounds Diet for a week (or less, if you reach your ideal weight before the completion of a week).

TO LOSE FIVE POUNDS OR LESS: Follow the Basic P-Type Weight Loss Diet for one week and then change to the P-Type Last Five Pounds Diet for a week (or less).

WHEN YOU REACH YOUR IDEAL WEIGHT: Change to the P-Type Health and Weight Maintenance Program.

Dishes marked with an asterisk are those for which a recipe is provided in Appendix 4.

THE BASIC PITUITARY TYPE WEIGHT LOSS DIET: GENERAL GUIDELINES

BREAKFAST

Choose either: 4 ounces of lean beef; 4 ounces of lean pork; 4 ounces of dark poultry meat; 4 ounces of lamb; 4 ounces of liver*; 4 ounces of kidney*; 4 ounces of heart*

Choose either: ½ cup of brown rice; ½ cup of bulghur wheat; ½ cup of millet; 1 cup of whole-grain cereal; 1 slice of whole-grain bread

1 cup of decaffeinated coffee, decaffeinated tea, or Fenugreek Tea

WAIT FOUR HOURS

LUNCH

Large green salad made with any combination of lettuce, cucumber, mushrooms, celery, sprouts, radishes, bell pepper, tomato or onion

1 teaspoon of clear diet dressing*

One 4 ounce serving of either beets, carrots, cauliflower, peas, potatoes, pumpkin or squash

4 ounces of shellfish or water-packed tuna

One piece of whole-grain bread

Choice of: 1 apple, 2 apricots, ½ banana, 1 cup of berries, ¼ cantaloupe, 10 cherries, 2 figs, ½ mango, 1 nectarine, 1 peach, 1 pear, ½ cup of pineapple, 2 plums, 1 cup of strawberries or 1 cup of watermelon

Fenugreek Tea

WAIT SIX HOURS

DINNER

Choice of either: 4 ounces of light poultry meat OR 4 ounces of fish or shellfish OR two eggs (three times a week only)

Fresh vegetables, steamed or raw, as much as you wish

One piece of fruit, same choices as lunch

Fenugreek Tea

THE BASIC P-TYPE WEIGHT LOSS DIET: A WEEK OF SAMPLE MENUS

MONDAY

BREAKFAST: 4 ounces of grilled calf's liver*
1 slice whole-wheat toast
Decaffeinated coffee

LUNCH: Large green salad with clear diet dressing*
4 ounces Broiled Shrimp with Lemon*
½ cup brown rice*
1 piece of fruit
Fenugreek Tea

DINNER: Stir-Fried Chicken* (or use a chicken recipe of your own, as long as you cook the chicken without the skin)
Baked apple (or other fruit in season)
Fenugreek Tea

TUESDAY

BREAKFAST: 4 ounces grilled lean minute steak
½ cup of brown rice*
Decaffeinated tea

LUNCH: Large green salad with clear diet dressing*
4 ounces broiled scallops
2 pieces of rye Krispbread
1 piece of fruit
Fenugreek Tea

DINNER: Celery-Onion Omelette* (or use your own egg recipe, using no more than 1 teaspoon of vegetable oil in cooking)

Steamed zucchini and string beans
Nectarine (or other fruit in season)
Fenugreek Tea

WEDNESDAY

BREAKFAST: 4 ounces broiled calf's liver*
                ½ cup millet*
                Decaffeinated coffee

LUNCH: Large green salad with clear diet dressing*
                4 ounces water-packed tuna with 1 teaspoon diet
                   mayonnaise
                1 slice of whole-grain bread
                1 piece of fruit
                Fenugreek Tea

DINNER: Chicken Breast* (or use a chicken recipe of your
                   own, preparing the chicken without skin)
                Steamed celery hearts
                1 cup of grapes (or other fruit in season)
                Fenugreek Tea

THURSDAY

BREAKFAST: Roasted Chicken Thigh (cooked in the oven the
                   night before with your Chicken Breast*)
                1 slice of whole-grain toast
                Decaffeinated coffee

LUNCH: Large green salad with clear diet dressing*
                4 ounces broiled shrimp
                ½ cup of brown rice*
                1 piece of fruit
                Fenugreek Tea

DINNER: Sole Provencal* (or use your own fish recipe, as
                long as fish is not breaded and you use 1
                teaspoon of vegetable oil only)

Poached Pear* (or other fruit in season)
Fenugreek Tea

FRIDAY

BREAKFAST: 4 ounces lean broiled pork chop
½ cup of bulghur wheat*
Decaffeinated tea

LUNCH: Large green salad with clear diet dressing*
4 ounces of broiled scallops
1 slice of rye bread
1 piece of fruit
Fenugreek Tea

DINNER: Lemon Chicken Kabobs with Mushrooms and
Zucchini* (or use your own chicken recipe,
using chicken without skin)
¼ cantaloupe (or other fruit in season)
Fenugreek Tea

SATURDAY

BREAKFAST: 4 ounces of broiled veal kidney*
½ cup of millet*
Decaffeinated coffee

LUNCH: Large green salad with clear diet dressing*
4 ounces of water-packed tuna with 1 teaspoon
diet mayonnaise
1 slice of whole-wheat toast
1 piece of fruit
Fenugreek Tea

DINNER: Stir-Fried Fish Fillets* (or use your own fish
recipe, as long as fish is not breaded and you
use only 1 teaspoon of vegetable oil)
1 cup of cherries (or other fruit in season)
Fenugreek Tea

SUNDAY

BREAKFAST: 4 ounces grilled lean minute steak
½ cup of brown rice*
Decaffeinated tea

LUNCH: Large green salad with clear diet dressing*
4 ounces of water-packed crab meat
2 pieces of rye Krispbread
1 piece of fruit
Fenugreek Tea

DINNER: Scrambled eggs with mushrooms
Stir-Fried Green Beans*
1 cup sliced fresh pineapple (or other fruit in season)
Fenugreek Tea

THE P-TYPE LAST
FIVE POUNDS
DIET

Remember, even if you have only five pounds of extra weight, you should not begin your P-Type Last Five Pounds Diet until you have followed the Basic P-Type Weight Loss Diet for a week. The sequence of diets is vital for balancing your metabolism, as well as for producing fast efficient loss of weight.

The P-Type Last Five Pounds Diet is a very special diet. It has about 1000 calories per day, about 200 calories per day less than the Basic P-Type Weight Loss Diet; and the food you eat is specially programmed to get you off the periodic plateaus of dieting, as well as to assist you in losing the stubborn last five pounds of excess weight. If you were to begin this diet at the start of your program you would probably find it difficult. But since you have been on the Basic P-Type Weight Loss Diet for at least a week, your metabolism is strengthened and in better balance, and you will be able to handle the Last Five Pounds Diet comfortably.

This diet is only to be followed for a week at a time. If, at the end of a week, you have not reached your ideal weight, return to the Basic P-Type Weight Loss Diet for one, two or three weeks, depending on your remaining extra weight. You may use the Last Five Pounds Diet every fourth week until you reach your weight goal. And as soon as you come within five pounds of your ideal weight, change to the Last Five Pounds Diet to lose that last bit of weight.

Note that the interval of time between meals has been increased on the Last Five Pounds Diet. Be sure to observe the full interval, as the hours between meals are the periods when your body is most active in burning fat.

THE P-TYPE LAST FIVE POUNDS DIET: GENERAL GUIDELINES

BREAKFAST

2 eggs, any style

1 teaspoon of vegetable oil

1 slice of whole-grain toast

1 cup of decaffeinated coffee or tea, or Fenugreek Tea (no sugar or honey)

WAIT FIVE HOURS

LUNCH

Choice of 1 apple or: 2 apricots, ½ banana, 1 cup of berries, ¼ cantaloupe, 10 cherries, 2 fresh figs, ½ mango, 1 nectarine, 1 peach, 1 pear, ½ cup of fresh pineapple, 2 plums, 1 cup of strawberries or 1 cup of watermelon.

Choice of either: 4 ounces of lean beef; 4 ounces of lean pork; 4 ounces of lamb; 4 ounces of dark poultry meat; 4 ounces of organ meat (liver, heart or kidneys)*

P-Type Vegetable Soup*, as much as you like

Fenugreek Tea

WAIT SIX HOURS

DINNER

4 ounces of fish or shellfish

1 slice of whole-grain bread

P-Type Vegetable Soup*, as much as you like

Fenugreek Tea

THE P-TYPE LAST FIVE POUNDS DIET: A WEEK OF SAMPLE MENUS

MONDAY

BREAKFAST: 2 eggs, any style
1 teaspoon of vegetable oil
1 slice of whole-grain toast
1 cup of decaffeinated coffee or tea, or Fenugreek Tea

LUNCH: Your choice of fruit
4 ounces of grilled lean hamburger
P-Type Vegetable Soup* (as much as you like)
Fenugreek Tea

DINNER: Baked Halibut Steak* (or use your own fish recipe, as long as fish is not breaded and you use only 1 teaspoon of vegetable oil)
1 slice of whole-grain bread
P-Type Vegetable Soup* (as much as you like)
Fenugreek Tea

TUESDAY

BREAKFAST: 2 eggs, any style
1 teaspoon of vegetable oil
1 slice of whole-grain toast
1 cup of decaffeinated coffee or tea, or Fenugreek Tea

LUNCH: Your choice of fruit
4 ounces grilled pork chop
P-Type Vegetable Soup* (as much as you like)
Fenugreek Tea

DINNER: Marinated Sole* (or use your own fish recipe, as
             long as fish is not breaded and you use only 1
             teaspoon of vegetable oil)
             1 slice of whole-grain bread
             P-Type Vegetable Soup* (as much as you like)
             Fenugreek Tea

WEDNESDAY

BREAKFAST: 2 eggs, any style
             1 teaspoon of vegetable oil
             1 slice of whole-grain toast
             1 cup of decaffeinated coffee or tea, or Fenu-
             greek Tea

LUNCH: Your choice of fruit
             4 ounces of dark-meat chicken
             P-Type Vegetable Soup* (as much as you like)
             Fenugreek Tea

DINNER: Stir-Fried Fish Fillet* (or use your own fish rec-
             ipe, as long as fish is not breaded and you use
             only 1 teaspoon of vegetable oil)
             1 slice of whole-grain bread
             P-Type Vegetable Soup* (as much as you like)
             Fenugreek Tea

THURSDAY

BREAKFAST: 2 eggs, any style
             1 teaspoon of vegetable oil
             1 slice of whole-grain toast
             1 cup of decaffeinated coffee or tea, or Fenu-
             greek Tea

LUNCH: Your choice of fruit
             4 ounces of grilled lamb chop
             P-Type Vegetable Soup* (as much as you like)
             Fenugreek Tea

DINNER: Salmon Steak Florentine* (or use your own fish recipe, as long as fish is not breaded and you use only 1 teaspoon of vegetable oil)
1 slice of whole-grain bread
P-Type Vegetable Soup* (as much as you like)
Fenugreek Tea

FRIDAY

BREAKFAST: 2 eggs, any style
1 teaspoon of vegetable oil
1 slice of whole-grain toast
1 cup of decaffeinated coffee or tea, or Fenugreek Tea

LUNCH: Your choice of fruit
4 ounces of grilled lean steak
P-Type Vegetable Soup* (as much as you like)
Fenugreek Tea

DINNER: Sole Provencal* (or use your own fish recipe, as long as fish is not breaded and you use only 1 teaspoon of vegetable oil)
1 slice of whole-grain bread
P-Type Vegetable Soup* (as much as you like)
Fenugreek Tea

SATURDAY

BREAKFAST: 2 eggs, any style
1 teaspoon of vegetable oil
1 slice of whole-grain toast
1 cup of decaffeinated coffee or tea, or Fenugreek Tea

LUNCH: Your choice of fruit
4 ounces of broiled liver*
P-Type Vegetable Soup* (as much as you like)
Fenugreek Tea

DINNER: Broiled Shrimp with Lemon* (or use your own
           shellfish recipe, using only 1 teaspoon of vege-
           table oil in preparation)
           1 slice of whole-grain bread
           P-Type Vegetable Soup* (as much as you like)
           Fenugreek Tea

SUNDAY

BREAKFAST: 2 eggs, any style
             1 teaspoon of vegetable oil
             1 slice of whole-grain toast
             1 cup of decaffeinated coffee or tea, or Fenu-
             greek Tea

LUNCH: Your choice of fruit
          4 ounces of grilled lean hamburger
          P-Type Vegetable Soup* (as much as you like)
          Fenugreek Tea

DINNER: Marinated Fish with Vegetables* (or use your
           own fish recipe, as long as fish is not breaded
           and you use only 1 teaspoon of vegetable oil)
           1 slice of whole-grain bread
           P-Type Vegetable Soup* (as much as you like)
           Fenugreek Tea

THE P-TYPE
HEALTH AND
WEIGHT
MAINTENANCE
PROGRAM

The formula for keeping the ideal weight you've achieved through your Body Type Diet is to have a continuing awareness of your body type and its special needs. Your P-Type Diet has brought about a state of balance in your metabolism; the P-Type Health and Weight Maintenance Program is designed to make it easy for you to *maintain* that balance, and to keep your ideal weight.

"PLENTY,"
"MODERATION" AND
"RARELY" FOODS

To make it as easy as possible for you to keep your body type requirements in mind, your program inclues a *short, simple* set of guidelines for your body type. You need only keep in mind: 1) your Plenty Foods (foods you can always eat, which will always be good for you); 2) your Moderation Foods (foods you can eat as long as you don't overdo them—I'll indicate your safe quantity of them), and 3) your Rarely Foods (ones you should save for special occasions only, because eating them will tend to revive your old cravings and make it harder for you to keep to your guidelines).

Continue to use your Herbal Tea and your Vegetable Soup. They will continue to strengthen your metabolism and are the best possible means for you to maintain the healthy balance you have achieved.

IF YOU FORGET THE
GUIDELINES AND GAIN
WEIGHT

If you stay with your guidelines you will not find yourself putting on weight. But if you let your guidelines go for any reason and you find yourself three to five pounds above your ideal weight, then go back to your original P-Type Weight Loss Program. With five extra pounds, you will need only a week of the P-Type Weight Loss Diet and a weekend of the P-Type Last Five Pounds Diet to be right back at your perfect weight.

THE P-TYPE HEALTH AND WEIGHT MAINTENANCE PROGRAM: GENERAL GUIDELINES

1. YOUR PLENTY FOODS: Beef, lamb and pork (without visible fat)
Organ meats: liver, kidneys, heart
Fresh vegetables, cooked or raw
Fenugreek Tea

2. YOUR MODERATION FOODS: Fruits
Whole Grains
Skim milk
Vegetable oils
Decaffeinated coffee and tea

3. YOUR RARELY FOODS: Yogurt
Ice Cream
Sour Cream
Cheese
Butter
Sugary desserts
Coffee, tea.

4. YOUR IDEAL EATING SCHEDULE: A substantial, protein-rich breakfast

A moderate lunch, with salad and some protein

A light dinner

Avoid late night eating

BREAKFAST

2 eggs, any style, OR a small minute steak, broiled, OR a slice of liver, kidneys or heart, broiled

1 slice of whole-grain bread

Decaffeinated coffee, tea or Fenugreek Tea

LUNCH

A large green salad with plenty of your favorite vegetables, and dressing used in moderation

2 slices of whole-grain bread, or an equivalent serving of other whole grains

A serving of fish, poultry or meat. You may substitute yogurt or cottage cheese *occasionally* (about every 2 weeks) if you feel good and are not overweight

1 piece of fruit

Decaffeinated coffee, tea or Fenugreek Tea

DINNER

A serving of fish, poultry or meat. Plan to eat meat 2-4 times a week, fish or poultry on the remaining nights

Vegetables, cooked or raw, as much as you like

1 glass of skim milk

1 piece of fruit, or a small dessert

Fenugreek Tea

10

MOST COMMONLY ASKED QUESTIONS ABOUT THE BODY TYPE DIET

QUESTION: *I don't understand why I need to know my body type. Isn't it true that if I eat fewer calories than I'm using up, I'll lose weight? Isn't all dieting just a matter of eating less?*

ANSWER: Yes, of course it is—in a sense. To lose weight you *must* take in fewer calories than your body burns. The physics of matter and energy haven't changed. But if you think about it, losing weight isn't all you want out of a diet. You want to lose weight *in the right places*. You want to look and feel great. And you want to keep off the weight you lose. Reaching these goals requires more than just any diet; it requires a diet that is right for your metabolism—that is, for your body type. If you need proof, just ask yourself how many diets you've been on before. Maybe you even lose weight on some of them. But was that enough? Somewhere they failed you. Your Body Type Diet won't.

QUESTION: *Is it possible to be a "mixed" body type? For example, could I be a mixed thyroid and adrenal type?*

ANSWER: No, not exactly. It is true that the exact proportion of strength of your four glands is unique to you, and that everyone has *some* characteristics of each type. But you always have one gland that is stronger than the other three, and so you do have one single body type.

Some people have well-balanced metabolisms in which the difference in activity among the four glands is not pronounced, but this is more often the case among slim people than among the overweight. The more overweight you are, the more likely you are to have a pronounced difference in the activity level of your glands—in other words, to be out of balance in your total metabolism.

Overweight is itself an unbalanced condition, and it is a chicken-and-the-egg question whether the glandular imbalance or the overweight comes first. People who rely a great deal on the energy of their dominant gland tend to overeat foods which stimulate that gland, setting up a cycle of imbalance that in turn promotes greater imbalance. The aim of the Body Type Diet is to reestablish balance among the glands: thus, as you lose weight, you will become less and less of a pronounced body type, and more and more of a balanced body type.

QUESTION: *Suppose I make a mistake in the Body Type Check List and decide I'm the wrong type. Will it hurt me to follow the diet for another type?*

ANSWER: All the Body Type Diets are healthy, balanced and nutritionally sound. They can't possibly hurt you. You'll even lose weight. It would be just as if you went to the bookstore and bought an ordinary, well-balanced "for-everyone" diet book.

What you won't get is the special benefits of a diet that's right for your body type. You won't get the reduction of foods which stimulate your dominant gland, and the extra support to build up your less active glands. That's the worst that can happen. But it's very unlikely to happen at all. The only way it might happen is if you are unable to look at yourself objectively, and the best way to avoid this possibility is to go through the Check List in Chapter 5 with a friend.

QUESTION: *A friend of mine lost a lot of weight on a high-protein diet, without knowing the first thing about body types. This shouldn't have happened, should it?*

ANSWER: Your friend is either a pituitary or a thyroid type. These two body types do fairly well on high-protein diets, although thyroid types often suffer from the caffeine drinks which most of these diets allow. Some people are lucky enough to find acceptable diets for their body types by accident. But even so, it will be to their advantage to know their body type, to understand how to keep off the weight they lost. The more knowledge we have about our bodies, the more intelligently we can care for them and maintain our weight and health.

QUESTION: *Doctor, what do you think about exercise? Will it help me on my body type diet?*

ANSWER: Exercise *is* good for you, but not for the reasons most people think. It can't do much by itself to help you lose weight. What it can do is maintain your skin and muscle tone *while you diet,* so that you arrive at your ideal weight in better condition.

Exercise, of course, does burn up calories, but it also gives you an excuse to eat more, so it's necessary to do a great deal of exercise before the calories it burns overbalances the resulting increase in appetite. Exercise reaches this level for most people when they are running about six miles per day, or the equivalent in other forms of activity. Most of us lack both the time and the inclination to exercise this much. A moderate exercise program—which I describe for you in Chapter 12—will make you feel better and look better, but it won't make you lose weight unless you also follow your Body Type Diet concurrently.

QUESTION: *I tend to eat a lot through nervousness. Is there anything I can do to relieve my tension and anxiety? So many times I think I'm eating for tension even though I'm not really hungry. And I get especially nervous when I'm dieting, because I know I'm not supposed to eat.*

ANSWER: For true relief of stress, there is no technique I have found to be more effective than Transcendental Meditation. It is a simple and easily learned technique and requires no particular belief or change in life style. As a doctor I have been impressed with the documented studies showing that 20 minutes of Transcendental Meditation, done twice a day, gives rest which is much deeper than sleep and relieves a wide range of physical and mental symptoms.

I practice TM regularly myself, and my experience bears out the scientific evidence. It is invariably refreshing and energizing. I have also found in patient after patient that those people who practice the Transcendental Meditation technique have a far easier time losing weight and keeping it off. This is undoubtedly because stress does play such a considerable role in overeating. Feeling rested and less stressed, people who meditate find they are far less likely to eat out of fatigue and tension.

To learn more about this valuable technique, I suggest you consult one of the many books on the subject, such as *The TM Book* by Denise Denniston and Peter McWilliams.

QUESTION: *Do you recommend a vitamin supplement with your Body Type Diet?*

ANSWER: If you've been taking vitamins and like them, there's no need to stop. But if you haven't, and feel all right without them, you don't need to start just because you are starting your Body Type Diet. The diets are balanced and nutritious, and don't cause any particular vitamin or mineral deficiency.

QUESTION: *Do I need to drink lots of extra water on my diet?*

ANSWER: You should be sure to drink all the liquids called for on your diet, especially the herbal teas. If you are thirsty between meals and want to drink additional water, fine, but you don't need to make a special effort to drink water if you aren't thirsty.

QUESTION: *I've heard some experts say that caffeine can interfere with weight loss, but other diet books say you can drink all you want. Personally, I can't think straight unless I've had a cup of coffee in the morning. Do I have to give it up to lose weight? What's the story, anyway?*

ANSWER: The ability to tolerate caffeine varies among the body types. Thyroid types must be very careful with caffeine, since it is so stimulating to the thyroid gland. Many T-types do indeed have to eliminate it to reach their ideal weight. Gonadal and adrenal types, by contrast, can actually benefit by the thyroidal stimulation it provides. They are allowed moderate amounts of caffeine in their Body Type Diets.

QUESTION: *Speaking of thyroid types, I'm an overweight T-type and I feel tired all the time. Doesn't that mean my thyroid is tired, and shouldn't I be taking thyroid pills?*

ANSWER: Supplementary thyroid is a medicine, and whether you need it or not can only be decided by your physician. In many overweight T-types there is some depression in the thyroid function, but I have found that in the majority of cases the Body Type Diet corrects the problem simply through elimination of thyroid-stimulating foods. Occasionally such a patient will need supplementary thyroid, but even when I do prescribe it I always retest the patient after a period on the diet. Usually the thyroid has revived and I can take the patient off thyroid pills. If you are taking thyroid pills, however, do not make the decision to stop on your own. Consult your doctor.

QUESTION: *What about salt and sugar? I've heard they're both terrible for you. Do your Body Type Diets eliminate them?*

ANSWER: Not necessarily. Again, like so many elements of diet, it depends upon your body type. Sugar and salt are both stimulating to certain glands, but the two substances create their effects in different ways. Sugar stimulates the thyroid, indirectly raises the blood glucose level and thus gives an immediate energy lift, while salt acts to contract the blood vessels and drive water out of the cells, causing a feeling of fullness and power. Thus the body types tend to use these substances in different ways. Pituitary and thyroid types eat sugar because they enjoy the feeling of quick energy, while adrenal and gonadal types are more apt to use salt for the powerful feeling it provides.

In my Body Type Diet, I use the effects of sugar and salt in a controlled way to offset certain tendencies of the body types. I allow a small amount of sugar to adrenal and gonadal types, who benefit from the thyroidal stimulation it provides. And I allow pituitary and thyroid types to have a small amount of salt with their foods, because the tightening of the system and the increased rigidity which salt produces counteract the tendency to vagueness and lack of focus which are characteristic of these types.

Certainly, sugar and salt in excess are harmful. I would not allow a patient of mine to have more than a small amount of either—but in small quantities these substances can be used with great benefit, provided the body type is taken into consideration.

QUESTION: *What about artificial sweeteners? Is it true they're bad for you?*

ANSWER: One thing is certain: they aren't foods. They can't possibly provide nourishment to the body in any way. The question, then, is whether they are harmful. The evidence at this point is not conclusive, but I am conservative and prefer to avoid risk. I don't recommend them.

QUESTION: *Doctor, do you recommend a diuretic? I sometimes feel so discouraged after dieting really strictly and not losing as much as I should because of water retention. This happens especially just before my period. Can I take a "water pill?"*

ANSWER: Some women, and a few men, do retain water for one reason or another. If you do, there are generally some medical implications, though they may not be serious. If you have a previously diagnosed condition for which your doctor has given you the OK to take a mild, over-the-counter diuretic, fine. Otherwise, you should see your doctor and find out why you're retaining water. Don't just start taking a diuretic on your own without having checked with your doctor first.

QUESTION: *I've been thinking of going on your Body Type Diet with my teenaged daughter, who is already a few pounds overweight. It is all right for a teenager to follow this diet?*

ANSWER: There is no problem at all, but it is wise to check with your doctor before starting a growing person on any diet. It's an excellent idea to acquaint your children with good eating habits for their body type. You can help them avoid many problems later on.

QUESTION: *Doctor, I'm pregnant but also overweight. Can I go on my Body Type Diet anyway?*

ANSWER: I feel, as do most doctors, that it's not a good idea to try to lose weight while pregnant. After you have your baby, by all means go on your Body Type Diet. In the meantime, follow your doctor's advice about diet. If you are only considering having a baby, keep in mind that the best situation is to get your body in balance through your Body Type Diet before you get pregnant, so that you'll have an easier pregnancy.

QUESTION: *What is your feeling about diet pills? Are they dangerous? Can they do any good?*

ANSWER: I believe that the best medicine is the least medicine. The body is a delicate mechanism, and all drugs have side effects in addition to their helpful qualities. The great majority of my patients feel so well on their Body Type Diet that they have no need for any medication; especially with the Snacking Strategy and the Herbal Teas for each type, hunger and cravings are rarely problems.

However, when it does happen that a patient asks me for a little bit of extra help, the type of pill I recommend depends on the body type. For pituitary and thyroid types, I use the bulk-filler pill; for adrenals and gonadals (when they need help, which is very rare), I use a diet pill of the amphetamine type in a carefully controlled dosage.

The two types of pills work in very different ways. The bulk-filler, as the name suggests, works by making the stomach feel full, so that you don't feel as much like eating. This type of pill sounds ideal, and would be if it only worked just a little bit better. Unfortunately, much of the time the reason we feel like eating has nothing to do with the stomach. It is more likely that we feel tense, fatigued or run down, and crave stimulation more than we crave a feeling of fullness in the stomach. These cravings are taken care of by the Body Type Diet, but if a P-type or T-type patient asks, I recommend this type of pill just until the diet takes hold.

The amphetamine-type pill, by contrast, works on the brain; it actually suppresses the idea of hunger, whether or not the body needs food. This type of pill should *never* be used by pituitary or thyroid types; it is far too stimulating. For adrenal and gonadal types, by contrast, amphetamine-type pills stimulate their thyroid somewhat, and can even help to balance their metabolism to a

limited extent. I sometimes prescribe them for a week or two,
until their diets are underway.

Some doctors may be shocked to hear that I occasionally
prescribe an amphetamine-type pill. In addition to their ability to
reduce hunger for a short time (that is, for a few weeks), these
pills also stimulate body and mind, and this property has given
these pills a history of abuse. However, having dealt with the
practical difficulties of weight control, as I have for many years,
I've learned that it's easy to tell a patient to lose weight and hand
him or her a diet; it's quite another to see overweight patients
keep their excess weight year after year because they can't get
started on a diet. My own feeling is that there is still a place for
amphetamine-type pills if they are used with a carefully designed
diet and under a doctor's supervision.

This is especially true with the more recently developed pills.
Because of the abuse factor, pharmaceutical companies have at-
tempted to reduce the stimulating effects of diet pills while retaining their hunger-suppressing qualities, with some success. A good
example is the drug Diethylpropion, an amphetamine-type pill
which can often be used even at night, since it causes no significant stimulation in many cases. Another example is Fenflura-
mine, an amphetamine-type pill which is actually a sedative to the
central nervous system. It is ocasionally prescribed by doctors
for very nervous patients who want to diet but need help controlling their hunger.

QUESTION: *Doctor, do you believe in fasting? I've always heard
it's the best way to lose weight, if you can only do it.*

ANSWER: Fasting has a strange fascination for dieters. I have
concluded that it is because food is such a problem to them; it
seems easier not to eat at all than to have to deal with eating
moderately and eating the right things. Yet fasting is not the
ultimate answer to weight control, since we must sooner or later
learn to eat properly to survive.

To the question of whether fasting is useful as a temporary
means of losing weight, my answer is yes, up to a point. I have
allowed many of my patients to fast for a couple of days—that is,
by abstaining from food but drinking fruit juice, vegetable juice or

broth. There is usually no problem in a one or two day fast for people in good health, though I do like to keep an eye on them.

However, there are problems with fasting. Deficiencies may develop, of vitamins, minerals or proteins, for example. Many people feel weak or irritable, or have headaches, while fasting, although some do not. It is even possible to do great harm to the body on extended fasts, if we fail to provide ourselves with some vital element that we need to keep on functioning.

On the other hand, I believe that the theory of fasting is sound, that by resting the entire machinery of digestion we give our bodies a chance to restore themselves more completely than they would ever be able to do normally.

The Last Five Pounds Diets for each body type provide what I consider to be an optimum balance between the values of fasting and its potential dangers. These diets are more restricted than the Weight Loss Diets, to the point where they can be considered as partial fasts. They "fast" the dominant gland by eliminating completely each body type's dominant gland stimulators; at the same time they provide nourishment for the less active glands, which relieves some of the negative side effects of fasting.

On the other hand, by allowing *some* food, the Last Five Pounds Diet has a positive value which total fasting lacks: that of helping you learn how to eat—how to handle food—so that once the fast is over you are not thrown back into the world of food as helpless as when you left it!

QUESTION: *Doctor, you say that your Last Five Pounds Diet helps get rid of cellulite. It sounds wonderful—I've got it and I hate it. But I read somewhere that there's no such thing—that it's only fat anyway. Is it really different from ordinary fat?*

ANSWER: Yes, it is. There are some diet "experts" who doubt the existence of cellulite, but I've seen too much of it—and seen how differently it behaves from ordinary fat—to say there's no such thing!

Of course, it looks different from ordinary fat. But more important is the internal difference. Cellulite gets its distinctive, wrinkly appearance by being more *toxic* than ordinary fat. That is, it contains more of the toxic by-products of faulty digestion, bad diet or illness than ordinary fat. This is what makes it so hard to lose.

When cellulite (or any fat, for that matter) is lost, it is burned up by the body, used as food. The body has more trouble using toxic fat. As thousands of dieters have told me, when they are losing toxic fat they actually feel toxic; that is, irritable, fatigued, weak—the negative feelings so often associated with dieting. These feelings make dieting so difficult that many dieters will simply stop dieting, preferring to keep the five extra pounds rather than go through the feelings involved in losing them.

I have designed the Last Five Pounds Diet for each type to combat the effects of losing toxic fat. The most important means is through the balancing of the metabolism which the entire Body Type Weight Loss Program provides. A more rested dominant gland, and strengthened support glands, handle the burning of cellulite much more effectively than the usual, weakened metabolism other diets produce.

Also, the Herbal Teas, the Snacking Strategy and above all the Vegetable Soups for each body type are designed to ease the process of digesting toxic fat. My patients tell me that they have so many strategies available to them for overcoming the "negatives" of dieting that, in fact, they never feel negative at all!

QUESTION: *What do you think about alcohol? Some diets let you drink white wine—or even liquor. What about yours?*

ANSWER: Mine doesn't. Alcohol has no place on a weight loss program. Not only does it add calories without adding nutritional value, it also makes you hungrier and less alert—which means less able to remember the principles of Body Type Dieting!

Of course, I know that even if they stop drinking for weight loss, many people enjoy alcohol and will continue to do so after they've reached their ideal weight. My caution would be that alcohol has a stimulating effect on the lower glands—the adrenals and gonadals—and that A-types and G-types are more susceptible to overdoing alcohol and putting on weight as a result.

QUESTION: *I know you don't recommend artificial sweeteners. But what about other "diet" foods—for instance, diet margarine, diet mayonnaise and diet salad dressings? Is there any harm in my eating them?*

ANSWER: My advice is to examine the individual product before buying it. In many "diet" foods the reduction in calories has been achieved, very simply, by adding water; this is the case with most diet margarines and mayonnaises. There is no harm in them, and they enable you to conserve calories while enjoying at least an approximation of the original food. You have to be careful about diet salad dressings, however. Many of them contain less calories than the equivalent nondiet dressing but are nevertheless quite calorie-laden; e.g. "diet" blue cheese dressings may contain forty calories per teaspoon—hardly a "diet" food. For this reason I specify that you use only *clear* diet dressings on your salad while on the Body Type Diet.

QUESTION: *Can laboratory tests be used to determine the body type? I think I'm a thyroid type, but I'd like to have a blood test of my thyroid levels to be sure that I'm right.*

ANSWER: Laboratory tests are neither necessary nor helpful in determining the body type. In the first place, they are unnecessary because the dominant gland shows itself so clearly in the way the body looks. I once had a patient who heard that I prescribed diet on the basis of the dominant gland, so she came to see me bearing a complete folder of lab tests she'd had done. She'd spent over one hundred dollars on the work. I looked at her without opening the folder and said that she was an adrenal type. I was sorry she'd spent that money; it was completely unnecessary.

Body shape is glandular chemistry writ large. The glands are like artists who work quietly in their studios behind the scenes, producing their works. The body is a work of art produced by all the glands together, masterminded by the dominant gland. Just as every artist has some characteristics by which his work can be recognized, so each of the glands has key characteristics which it imparts to bodies it dominates. As a result, every individual has distinguishing features that point to his or her dominant gland. Once you know what to look for, you will be able to read these marks as easily as I can.

In the second place, using lab tests to find blood hormone

levels is not as simple as it sounds. There is a great deal of fluctuation in hormone levels in the body, both on a daily basis and in the course of longer cycles, such as the menstrual cycle. A "high" level of pituitary hormone and a "low" level of a female sex hormone at any given time would not necessarily indicate a pituitary type; it might just as well indicate a particular point in a woman's monthly cycle.

QUESTION: *I am definitely a thyroid type—I have all the characteristics. But I've had my thyroid level tested for other reasons, and I know it's very low. How can I be a thyroid type when I have such a low level of thyroid function?*

ANSWER: This is a common occurrence. In the overweight, the dominant gland may be slightly subnormal—that is, a little depressed in its functioning. The depression of the gland is due to overstimulation and subsequent exhaustion.

The glands do not all become exhausted at the same rate; the thyroid gland becomes overtired quite easily, while the adrenals are much harder to exhaust. The gonads and the pituitary fall between these two extremes. For this reason the situation is most common in thyroid types, and least common in adrenal types.

The Body Type Diet usually takes care of the exhaustion of the thyroid, and supplementary hormones are not needed unless there are also medical problems with the gland itself.

QUESTION: *I have gone through the Body Type Check List and have no doubt about which body type I am. But I don't have the cravings I ought to have. I'm a G-type, but what I crave is sweets. What does this mean?*

ANSWER: It means that the cravings natural to your body type have been supressed and another set of cravings substituted. This doesn't happen often, but it does happen—and there is one big reason why it does.

The reason is early conditioning. There are some families and some cultures which emphasize a particular food group very strongly. For example, there are families who insist on having meat at every meal, and who tell the children how healthy, nourishing, nonfattening, and generally desirable meat is. People from such a background sometimes develop a craving for meat even if they are thyroid or pituitary types, but the craving is mostly psychological rather than physical.

In the same way, some families emphasize sweets heavily. This must have been your case. Since sugar does have such a strong thyroid-stimulating quality, and since everyone, after all, has a thyroid gland, it is possible for people of any body type to develop a "sweet tooth" on the basis of early conditioning. Again, it is not *common* for this to happen to an adrenal or gonadal type—but it can.

It would be more common than it is, except for the fact that most of us have psychological associations with many types of food. Naturally we tend to select our cravings from the foods that correspond to our body type. Two patients—a brother and sister—illustrate how this works. They came from a warm Italian-American family, and both were deeply attached to the foods of their childhood. But the brother, a thyroid type, was attracted mainly to the pasta—a typical T-type craving. The sister, by contrast, who was a gonadal type, all but dreamed of the spicy sausage dishes her mother used to make. Both had selected, from the identical background, foods which were stimulating to their dominant gland. They told me they had spent their childhood finishing what was on each other's plates!

However, since psychological factors sometimes intrude on body-type cravings, I do not use cravings as an absolute guide to body type. I always give emphasis to the body shape. While cravings and body type will correspond ninety percent of the time, body shape is a one hundred percent reliable guide to body type.

QUESTION: *Doctor, I've tried to go through the Body Type Check List but I am more than fifty pounds overweight and I can't seem to distinguish my body shape. I've lost my shape everywhere. I'm ready to diet, but how do I find my body type?*

ANSWER: What you have to do is to look beneath your extra weight to find your body type. One way to do this is to study pictures of yourself when you were less overweight. Another way is to get the help of someone who knew you when you were slimmer, or to consult your own memory. Then go through the Body Type Check List answering the questions *as you were then*. Your body type does not change, so the type you were then is the type you are now. Good luck! I know you will succeed with your Body Type Diet.

11

EATING OUT
ON THE BODY
TYPE DIET

Eating out does *not* have to mean the end of your Body Type Diet!
By keeping the principles of eating for your body type firmly in
mind, you can enjoy a meal out and not lose ground while you're
dieting. You can even lose weight!

Of course, the degree of control you have over your food
varies when you eat out. The range is all the way from a restaurant
you select yourself with your body type in mind, to dinner at the
home of a friend or relative who has selected the menu in accor-
dance with needs of her own. This is an area in which life is
compromise; do the best you can, and resolve to go back to your
Body Type Diet at the very next meal.

FOR ALL BODY
TYPES TO KEEP IN
MIND:

PLAN AHEAD. Before going out to eat in a restaurant, take a
moment to think about what you will eat. Review the "Plenty
Foods" and "Moderation Foods" in your Body Type Health
and Weight Maintenance Program, and plan your meal to in-
clude lots of Plenty Foods and one or two Moderation Foods. If
you have thought through your eating plan, you will have less
trouble resisting the danger foods for your body type.

ORDER A SALAD FIRST. You can save yourself many calories by
ordering a big salad as your first course. Ask for oil and vinegar
dressing to be brought to the table, then skip the oil and just use
the vinegar—or ask for fresh lemon to squeeze over the salad.
By the time you've enjoyed your salad you'll have taken the

edge off your hunger, and can eat moderately and happily according to your eating plan.

BRING A TEABAG OF YOUR BODY TYPE HERBAL TEA. It's smart always to carry several teabags with you in your purse or briefcase. Ask for hot water and make yourself a cup of your tea. It will soothe your body and revive your will power instantly!

EAT SLOWLY. A restaurant meal is a treat and should be enjoyed; the more you enjoy the food you order, the less it will take to satisfy you. In a fast-food restaurant, you can buy fast food but you don't have to *eat* it fast. Sit down, eat and appreciate. Focus on the food for maximum pleasure from minimum calories.

DRINK WATER AT THE TABLE. It's surprising how much of what we think is desire to eat is actually compounded of thirst and the need to do *something* with our mouths. Having a glass of water to sip is a major way to avoid constant eating.

GUIDELINES FOR GONADAL TYPES

YOUR WORST TEMPTATION in a restaurant is spicy dishes, which will stimulate your appetite and make you lose control over your eating. The strategy to avoid it: carry a piece of fruit with you and eat it just before you leave for the restaurant. The fruit will help balance your system so that resisting spicy foods becomes easier, not harder. In any case it is psychologically difficult to eat spicy foods after cool, fresh fruit.

YOUR BEST ORDER for your main course is fish. Ask that it be broiled or baked. Chicken is also an acceptable choice, but be careful of barbecued chicken, because the sauce is too salty and spicy for you. Avoid red meat and casserole-type dishes (e.g. Beef Stroganoff), which are made with creamy sauces. Also avoid most ethnic dishes (Mexican, Indian, etc.)—again, too spicy. In Chinese restaurants, do not select a Hunan or Szechwan-style dish. Choose Cantonese-style dishes based on chicken, fish and vegetables. Remember, Chow Mein is the one with noodles and Chop Suey is mainly vegetables. Obviously, Chop Suey is for you.

IN A FAST-FOOD RESTAURANT, be aware that the main problem for you is the excessive oil used in cooking. In a hamburger place, the trick is to order a fish sandwich, remove the tartar sauce, throw away the top piece of bread, and blot the fish with your napkin. Don't order fries. Some fast-food places have a salad bar; if available, a big salad is your best bet. Another good choice for fast food for you: frozen yogurt. Avoid pizza restaurants and Mexican-style fast food (too spicy).

GUIDELINES FOR ADRENAL TYPES

YOUR WORST TEMPTATION in a restaurant is to order a big steak with salad and make believe you had a healthy diet meal. Have the salad, but with tuna fish or cottage cheese instead. Before-meal appetizers (peanuts, salty snacks) are also a temptation for you, so if these are on the table in a restaurant ask that they be taken away *immediately,* before you have a chance to weaken. If you eat one, you'll eat a lot of them. Drinks can also be a temptation. Order a club soda or mineral water, with a twist of lemon for eye and taste appeal. If you simply can't resist a drink, the *only* acceptable choice is a wine spritzer— white wine mixed with club soda. Sip it slowly and make it last.

YOUR BEST ORDER for a main dish is breast of chicken or turkey, but be sure to request that it is baked or broiled, not fried. The classic "dieter's plate" in many restaurants consists of fruit, cottage cheese and a hamburger patty; this is a good choice for you if you ask them to leave off the hamburger. Fruit salad with cottage cheese is another good choice at either lunch or dinner.

IN A FAST FOOD RESTAURANT, the main thing to avoid is the hamburger. Look for something without red meat—for example, a chicken taco or a mostly lettuce burrito in a Mexican-style place. A slice of *cheese* (not meat) pizza once in a while is acceptable, though it is too salty for you to make a habit of it. In a hamburger restaurant, a fish sandwich is a possible choice. Or you can have frozen yogurt with a granola topping. For really fast food, carry a covered mug full of granola with you and order a carton of milk to pour over it—perfect for your body type.

GUIDELINES FOR
THYROID TYPES

YOUR WORST TEMPTATION in a restaurant comes right at the beginning—the bread on the table. The best strategy is to ask to have it taken away immediately, *before* you start to nibble on it. Then order a seafood cocktail right away—the protein in the shrimp or crab will strengthen your body and your will power by keeping your thyroid gland cooled off.

YOUR BEST ORDER for a main dish in a restaurant is broiled or baked chicken. An omelette is another good entree if you did not have eggs for breakfast. At the end of the meal, if you've eaten a good, high-protein entree, you'll be in a good position to resist your second major temptation, dessert. If you feel you may not be able to resist, excuse yourself and go to the bathroom while the others at your table are ordering dessert. Then, while the others eat, call for hot water and make your Raspberry Leaf Tea. You may order the cheese plate for dessert if you wish, but if it comes with fruit, restrict yourself to half an apple at most. Avoid the bowl of mints at the cash register by having someone else pay the bill.

IN A FAST FOOD RESTAURANT, you are in relatively good shape, since protein foods are readily available. A hamburger or a chicken or fish sandwich are all acceptable—as long as you throw away the bread and blot the meat with your napkin. Also, many places have a variation of Eggs Benedict, consisting of an egg with a slice of meat and cheese. Again, throw away the bread and have the rest. In some fast-food restaurants certain specialty sandwiches are served on whole-wheat bread. If you find one like this, you only have to throw away the *top* piece of bread; you may eat the bottom piece. You may be tempted by a cola drink, but you *must* resist. The best strategy for this is to order water—all restaurants will gladly supply you with a cup of it. Drink it right away; if you're not thirsty, your temptation to drink a cola will be much less. Caffeine-free diet sodas are also a possibility occasionally.

GUIDELINES FOR PITUITARY TYPES

YOUR WORST TEMPTATION in a restaurant is to order something with cheese on it—a cheeseburger, or anything *au gratin*—with cheese. Your best strategy to avoid this is to order something high-protein immediately—for example, a shrimp cocktail. The protein will help you feel strong enough to resist those cheesy, creamy dishes that no P-type would dream of making at home, but that always seem to appear on restaurant menus. Another temptation for you: the desire to eat a heavy meal at night when dining out. Avoid it by concentrating on protein.

YOUR BEST ORDER in a restaurant is a shrimp or crab salad, or an omelette. Stay away from dishes with sauces—they are invariably too creamy for your metabolism. In a really elegant restaurant? Order Steak Tartare—raw chopped meat with seasonings. Perfect for you! In a Japanese restaurant, have raw fish, not sushi (too much rice) or tempura (too greasy).

IN A FAST FOOD RESTAURANT, order a hamburger (but not a cheeseburger). Throw away the top piece of the roll and blot the burger with a napkin—twice. No shakes for you, ever—and no cola drinks while you are dieting. Request a cup of water, or ask for hot water and make Fenugreek Tea. Stay away from pizza places—no pizza has ever agreed with a pituitary type. In a Mexican-style restaurant, skip the enchiladas (they have melted cheese on the top). If you order a taco, be sure to request that they leave off the grated cheese. Fast-food rotisseried chicken is acceptable once in a while *if* you pull off the skin before you eat it.

12

THE BODY
TYPE
EXERCISE
PROGRAM

Much research has been devoted to exercise in the last few years, especially on the relationship between exercise and longevity. Studies have focused particularly on finding out whether exercise prevents heart attacks and other cardiovascular diseases. Researchers have also tried to determine the value of exercise in weight control. The subject of exercise and heart disease remains open—the results of research are not yet final. But on the subject of weight control, research has confirmed what many people have found out for themselves: an exercise program by itself is *not* of great value in losing weight.

This does not mean that you do not need to exercise—far from it. But it does mean that exercise should be put into perspective in the context of Body Type Dieting.

There are many reasons why people exercise, the most common being to lose weight, to improve their health, and simply to blow off steam and unwind from the pressures of the day. The last reason is probably the most common. Exercise puts the mind at rest while the body is given a workout, and this change brings relief. The exercise period also provides a time to oneself, free of other people's demands. It frees us, for a time, from the stress of normal daily living.

On the other hand, many people who exercise to reduce stress also eat to reduce stress—and most people eat back the calories they expended jogging or working out. This is why exercise alone, without an accompanying diet program that is right for your body type, will not result in loss of weight. If the exercise is enjoyable and provides a break in routine, that is enough to ask of it.

Exercise does burn up calories, but it's necessary to exercise a great deal before the calories expended become truly significant and begin to outweigh the increase in appetite that exercise also produces. To reach this level most people need to run about six miles per day, or its equivalent in some other form of strenuous activity. Few of us have either the time or the inclination to exercise this much. For those of us who exercise more moderately, the calories expended are not enough to produce weight loss without also following the Body Type Diet.

But what about the reduction of stress that exercise is supposed to give? Again, the fact is that exercise cannot accomplish this goal. The key to reducing stress (which may be defined as the accumulated fatigue of our activity, which may be mental, physical or emotional) is not further activity but *rest*. Obviously, we cannot be at rest and exercising at the same time, and we should not expect to accomplish the goals of rest and activity at once. If you wish to rid yourself of the fatigue of a stressful day, what you need is a period of deep rest.

Fatigue, stress and tension have results in the body which are similar to disease. These effects are the opposite of energetic good health, which can be restored only by rest. Exercise gives us a break from a certain kind of mental stress, but it cannot get *rid* of the stress—only take our attention away from it for a time. The truth is that to *cure* stress and fatigue, we must turn to something that gives rest.

For this, I recommend the technique of Transcendental Meditation. I have already explained, in Chapter 10, the value of Transcendental Meditation in controlling "nervous eating"—eating which is due to stress. But the benefits of Transcendental Meditation, or TM, go beyond this kind of help to a general and very beneficial reduction in stress throughout the entire system. Research has shown that TM also increases our ability to deal with difficult situations, so that stress does not build up as rapidly in the first place. For general relief of stress, then, the practice of Transcendental Meditation is incomparably preferable to exercise.

This leaves us, finally, with only one important reason for exercising: to improve our physical health and vitality. And here—rather than for weight control or for stress reduction—we find the true value of exercise. Though research is still studying the question, there are a number of indications that exercise will help us to live longer, feel better, and be less prone to many diseases.

The true purpose of exercise is to build up physical strength. Exercise maintains muscle tone, increases physical energy, and makes you feel good all over. For all these reasons, exercise has a very definite place in a program for maintaining total health in today's fast-paced environment.

The question then becomes how you can decide on the ideal exercise program for yourself. So many patients have asked me to help them with this question that I have designed four separate exercise programs, for the special needs of the four body types. Just as the body types have different metabolic styles, they have different exercise styles as well. An exercise program can accomplish a great deal if it is chosen with the body type in mind.

The right exercise program for your body type can supplement the effects of diet in *balancing* the metabolism, help in *removing* fat that accumulates in especially stubborn spots on each body type, and assist in *strengthening* the dominant gland, which as you know is tired and overworked in the overweight.

To accomplish these goals, the Body Type Exercise Program has three parts. First, there's a Total Body Exercise for each body type, chosen both for its value in giving a workout to the cardiovascular system and for its effects in balancing the metabolism of the body type (I'll explain how this works for each body type as I describe the exercises).

Second, each type has a set of Spot-Toning Exercises, which work directly on the area of that body type where stubborn fat is always found. And third, there is a Body Position, taken from the tradition of Yoga positions, for each body type. I have chosen Body Positions for their value in strengthening each body type's dominant gland.

Since you already know your body type, you need only select the Body Type Exercise Program that is right for you. To take full advantage of the benefits, do fifteen to twenty minutes of your Total Body Exercise three times a week. Do the Spot-Toning Exercises and the Yoga Position every day; they will take no more than five or ten minutes.

If you have not exercised before, or are in poor condition or very overweight, you should have a complete physical examination by a doctor before beginning this or any other exercise program. Even if you have been active in the past, you should never begin exercising suddenly. Work up to the full program by starting to do your Total Body Exercise with only five minutes three times a week. Increase after a week to ten minutes three times a week. Then after another week you may increase to fifteen minutes three times a week.

Patients have also asked me if the Body Type Exercise Program is necessary for loss of weight The answer is no. It isn't strictly necessary; your Body Type Diet works well by itself. If you have energy only for one self-improvement program, your Body Type Diet is the more important change for you as an overweight person than the Exercise Program. However, if you wish to start both simultaneously, I certainly encourage you to do so.

THE GONADAL-TYPE EXERCISE PROGRAM

THE GONADAL-TYPE TOTAL BODY EXERCISE is designed, in addition to toning the cardiovascular system, to improve grace and balance and to integrate mental processes with physical energy.

As a G-type you have plenty of bodily awareness, but your metabolism receives a balancing effect when you do exercises that involve the mind intimately with the body. By choosing exercises that involve thought, such as martial arts exercises or dance, you integrate your awareness of your body more fully into the total structure of your personality.

For this reason I recommend for G-types martial arts such as Kung Fu or karate, ballet, or jazz dancing. Choose one of these exercises and do it three times a week for fifteen to twenty minutes; or enjoy the variety of doing more than one if you prefer.

THE GONADAL-TYPE SPOT-TONING EXERCISES are all focused on your danger areas—mainly the rear end, but also the thighs and upper hips. Do each one every day.

1. REAR END WALK: Sit on the floor, legs stretched out in front of you. "Walk" on your hips, forward five steps, back five steps. Start with one repetition, gradually increase to five.

2. LEG LIFT: Get on your hands and knees; stretch one leg out behind you. Raise the leg until it is straight out behind you; lower to the floor. Change and repeat with the other leg. Start with five "lifts" on each leg, and gradually increase to fifteen.

3. LEG CIRCLES: Lie flat on your back, arms out at sides. Bend one knee and put that foot on the floor in front of you. Raise the other leg towards the ceiling. Make a wide circle with it, bringing it down towards the floor all around but not touching the floor. Then change position and repeat with the other leg. Start with five "circles" with each leg, and gradually increase to ten.

4. SIDE-TO-SIDE ROLL: Sit on the floor, legs stretched out in front of you, hands on the floor slightly behind your body. Keeping your legs straight, roll over onto one hip while raising the opposite arm. Then roll back onto the other hip, lowering the raised arm and leaning your weight on it. Each time you roll, raise the opposite arm over your head and stretch it towards the ceiling. Start with five "rolls" and gradually increase to twenty.

5. FANNY HOLDS: Lie on the floor, face down, with a pillow or rolled towel under your stomach. Draw your buttocks together as tightly as possible. Hold. Then release the muscles gradually. Start with five "holds," gradually increasing to ten.

THE GONADAL-TYPE BODY POSITION should be done every day after the Spot-Toning Exercises. Lie on the floor, face down. Place your hands, in fists, under your hips. Slowly raise one leg into the air. Hold for three to five seconds, then lower the leg to the floor. Repeat with the other leg, and hold three to five seconds. *Do not strain;* raise each leg only as high as is comfortable. After doing this position for several months, if it becomes very easy to do, you may begin raising both legs at the same time, and holding three to five seconds. Then turn onto your back and rest in this position for two or three minutes. The G-type Body Position, with the brief rest, is very strengthening to the sex glands.

THE ADRENAL-
TYPE EXERCISE
PROGRAM

THE ADRENAL-TYPE TOTAL BODY EXERCISES is designed to encourage your body to develop quickness and flexibility. The A-type metabolism has no lack of power, but can benefit from exercises involving eye-hand coordination and quick, precise movements.

The exercises that accomplish this most effectively are tennis, ballet, jazz dancing, or racketball. Doing one or all of these exercises on a regular basis—at least fifteen or twenty minutes three times a week—will spontaneously bring about a balancing of your metabolic activity.

THE ADRENAL-TYPE SPOT-TONING EXERCISES are designed to help tone and reduce your danger areas: waist, abdomen, upper arms and breasts. Do each one every day.

1. CROSSOVERS: Lie on the floor on your back, arms extended above your head. Keeping your back flat on the floor, raise your right arm and left leg, touching your hand to the knee. *Do not strain;* go only as far as is comfortable. Then return your leg to the floor and your arm to its original position over your head. Press your arm gently to the floor. Relax. Repeat with the other arm and leg. Begin with five crossovers with each leg, and gradually increase until you are doing fifteen with each leg.

2. BUTTERFLIES: Lie on your back, knees bent, feet flat on the floor, arms at your sides. Keeping your arms flat on the floor, slide them upwards to shoulder level. Press your back towards the floor. Continue to slide your arms upwards until they are over your head. Again, press back to the floor. Slide the arms back to your side, stopping again at shoulder level to press your back to the floor. Start with three "butterflies" and increase until you are doing six.

3. ARM CIRCLES: Stand with your feet slightly apart and your arms extended outward at shoulder level. Make six-inch circles with both hands in the air. Do five circles clockwise, then reverse and go counterclockwise. Gradually increase until you can do ten circles in each direction.

4. OVERHAND STRETCHES: Stand with your feet apart and hands on your hips. Raise your right arm over your head, then stretch it over your head and towards the opposite side. Stretch your waist and bend your upper body towards the left side as you reach with your arm. Stretch three times with the right arm, then change and stretch towards the right side with your left arm. Start by doing this once to each side, and increase until you are doing five triple "stretches" to each side.

THE ADRENAL-TYPE BODY POSITION should be performed each day after you have finished your Spot-Toning Exercises. Sit on the floor with your legs straight out in front of you. Stretch your arms out towards your feet. Slowly bend your body forward until you are as close as you can get to touching your toes with your fingers. If you can touch your toes, bend forward even more and bring your upper body down towards your thighs. Go *only as far as you can comfortably;* do not strain. Hold the position for three to five seconds. Then slowly straighten up and lie down on your back for two or three minutes. The combination of the position with the rest is highly strengthening to the adrenal glands.

THE THYROID-TYPE EXERCISE PROGRAM

THE THYROID-TYPE TOTAL BODY EXERCISE is designed to provide what the thyroid-type metabolism needs most: endurance. The up-and-down quality of your metabolism is its principal weakness, since it is very apt to give rise to overeating of thyroid-stimulating foods during periods of fatigue.

This weakness of the T-type metabolism can be eliminated completely through a combination of diet and exercise. I have chosen exercises for you which give a workout to your entire body in a sustained way. These exercises also will improve circulation and help your tissues make better use of your thyroid hormone.

The Total Body Exercises which are most effective in providing these values, with the most value for thyroid types, are swimming, jogging and aerobic dancing. Doing one or a variety of these exercises regularly will bring about additional balancing of the T-type metabolism.

THE THYROID-TYPE SPOT-TONING EXERCISES focus on your danger areas: outer thighs and midriff roll. Do each exercise every day.

1. SITUPS: Lie on your back on the floor with legs slightly apart and your arms extended over your head. In one continuous motion, swing arms up and bring yourself to a sitting position. Then bend forward and reach for the floor between your legs. *Don't force;* go only as far as is comfortable. Slowly lower your body to the floor, rolling your back as you go. Rest for a moment on the floor and then repeat. If the exercise is very difficult, start by hooking your feet under the edge of a couch or bed to hold them. After doing situps for several weeks you will no longer need your feet held. Start with two or three situps and increase gradually until you are doing ten each day.

2. LEG CIRCLES: Lie flat on your back, arms out at sides. Bend one knee and put that foot on the floor in front of you. Raise the other leg towards the ceiling. Make a wide circle with it, bringing it down towards the floor all around but not touching the floor. Then change position and repeat with the other leg. Start with five "circles" with each leg, and gradually increase to ten.

3. TOE TOUCHERS: Stand with feet apart and hips tucked under. Extend your arms out from your shoulders. Bend and reach your right hand towards your left toe—making sure to *bend* your knees. (If you keep your knee locked straight you may strain your back.) Straighten up and bend again, reaching with your left hand towards your right toe. Start with four "touchers" to each side and gradually increase until you are doing ten to each side.

4. MIDRIFF ROLLS: Lie on your back, arms out at your sides at shoulder level. Draw your legs up to your chest. Keeping knees together, let both your knees fall to the right side. Then pull them up again towards your chest. Repeat to the other side. Start with five rolls to each side, gradually increasing until you are doing ten to each side.

THE THYROID-TYPE BODY POSITION should be done each day after you finish your Spot-Toning Exercises. Lie flat on your back on the floor. Slowly raise your legs until they are over your body. Then, supporting your back with your hands, raise your hips and back until they are vertical over your shoulders (see drawing). Hold the position for three to five seconds. Slowly lower your body to the floor; then lower your legs. After doing the position, lie and rest for two or three minutes. When doing the position, take it very easy and do not strain. If you cannot reach the full position, go *only as far as is comfortable*. As you diet and continue with your exercise program, you will find the position becoming easier until you can do it without difficulty. The combination of this Body Position and the rest is very strengthening to the thyroid gland.

THE PITUITARY-
TYPE EXERCISE
PROGRAM

THE PITUITARY-TYPE TOTAL BODY EXERCISE has been chosen with two purposes in mind, corresponding to the needs of your pituitary-type metabolism. The first is to increase your awareness of your body. As you know, the Pituitary-Type Weight Loss Diet works to increase your bodily awareness by stimulating your lower glands—the adrenals and the gonads. The P-Type Total Body Exercise helps accomplish this by involving your lower body in the exercise as much as possible.

The second purpose is to increase stimulation to the adrenals. Again, stimulating the adrenals is the most effective way to produce balance in your metabolism. Exercises which specifically develop your large muscles (weight lifting, calesthenics) stimulate the adrenal glands directly.

The Total Body Exercises that are most effective for these purposes are weight lifting, calesthenics, hiking, backpacking, or horseback riding. Choose one and do it regularly, or do all of them for variety, as long as you do one of them for at least fifteen minutes three times a week.

THE PITUITARY-TYPE SPOT-TONING EXERCISES go after your danger areas for fat accumulation—chest, stomach, and knees. Do them for five to ten minutes every day to keep these areas firm and fat-free.

1. BICYCLING: Lie on the floor, face up, arms out at your sides. Support your lower back with a pillow or a rolled-up towel. Draw up your knees towards your chest. Straighten one leg towards the ceiling, then bring it back towards your chest and straighten the other leg, as if you were riding a bicycle in the air. A circle of both legs counts as one repetition. Start with ten "cycles" and gradually increase to fifty over a period of two weeks.

2. SIDEWAYS BICYCLING: Lie on the floor on your side. Raise both legs just off the floor. Bend and straighten each leg in

turn, as if riding a bicycle. Count each revolution of both legs as one repetition. Begin with ten "cycles" and gradually increase to twenty-five. After you have been doing this exercise for some time and if it becomes easy, you can increase its effect by raising your upper body off the floor and supporting it on your bent arms.

3. UPPER BODY STRETCHES: Lie on your back on the floor, knees bent, and extend your arms above your head. Press your back to the floor at the waist. Stretch up first one arm, and then the other over your head. Really stretch. Hold each "stretched" position for a few seconds, then relax and change to the other arm. Begin with three times for each arm, and gradually increase to six times with each arm.

4. BUST SQUEEZES: Sit on the floor or in a chair, whichever is comfortable. Extend your arms at shoulder level and bring your palms together in front of you. Press the heels of your hands together. Hold this position for several seconds, and then relax. Start with five "squeezes" and gradually increase to ten.

THE PITUITARY-TYPE BODY POSITION should be done after you have finished your Spot-Toning Exercises each day. Sit on the floor with legs crossed, tailor style. Lie down, still with legs crossed. Raise your arms over your head and place your palms on the floor. Pushing with your palms, gently arch your back and neck until the top of your head rests on the floor, being careful to support your weight on your palms, not on your head (see drawing). Hold this position for five seconds. Then gently lower your back and neck to the floor. After doing the position, rest, lying on the floor, for two or three minutes. The combination of the Body Position and the rest, performed every day, is extremely strengthening to the pituitary gland.

13

HEALTH, LONGEVITY, AND WEIGHT CONTROL

Our discussion of weight control has taken us a long way. Starting from the problem of why diets work for some people and not for others, we've looked deeply into the way the metabolism works in each of four body types. You've found which body type yours is, and learned how you can use food to support your body's strengths and eliminate its weaknesses. You've seen how you can bring about the state of positive and healthy glandular balance that will enable you to reach, and maintain, your ideal weight.

The Body Type Diet has been constructed to help you make maximum use of your body's inborn potential for health, vitality and long life. The particular diet for each body type not only takes off weight—which many diets, both good and bad, will do, at least temporarily—but actually *transforms* your body permanently. The days of reshaping the flesh without giving a thought to health are, fortunately, gone. Today, physicians and dieters alike think in terms of beauty which comes from underlying good health, and not in terms of a cosmetic improvement achieved at any cost.

Even styles in clothing reflect this changed attitude. For modern women, the girdle is a thing of the past, replaced by a positive shapeliness brought about by diet and exercise. I am convinced that this change represents an increased understanding that health and beauty are the same thing, and that what is seen on the surface can only reflect the quality of what is within.

The body is in a perpetual state of change. It is often said that every cell in the body is changed every seven years, but the truth is that most areas of the body change far more quickly than that. If every cell is in a state of change, the food we eat must always be of the highest quality, in order to be sure that change results in positive transformation, day after day and year after year.

In structuring the diets I have always considered which parts of the body are, in each body type, in most urgent need of support and repair. If the thyroid gland is weak and tired, the diet must contain food which will assist the body in its efforts to repair that gland. If the adrenal gland has been overstimulated, the diet must be designed to rest the adrenals and must contain materials with which they can be restored. In every case, the diet is designed to assist the body in its constant process of self-transformation.

If a car breaks down, we can always put it into the shop and get the repairs done. But with our bodies, the processes of life must continue while the repairs are being made. When you go on a diet, you are in effect doing on-the-road repairs on your body. Specifically, you are deciding to devote more energy to repair, restructuring and rebuilding than is usual in your daily life. Whenever you eat less than you need to maintain a constant weight, you are involved in some restructuring of your body, so it is vitally important that any weight-loss diet take into account this aspect of bodily transformation, while continuing to provide nourishment for the ongoing processes of life itself.

When the transformation of the Body Type Diet is complete, you will feel better than you ever felt before. Ideal weight, as defined in the context of Body Type Dieting, is synonymous with perfect health. If your body were to show the right weight on the scales, and yet you were tired all the time, or had trouble sleeping, or were subject to frequent colds or other annoying small illnesses, then you would *not* be at your ideal weight, no matter what the scales might say. You could be skinny as a rail, but the stuff of your body would not be the right stuff. Your ideal weight is the one at which you look and feel your best, at which your energy is steady and strong and you enjoy the health and vitality that are your birthright as a human being.

Ideal weight cannot be separated from quality of life. And from quality of life naturally flows longevity, length of life. Life continues to flourish on the basis of continual transformation. As long as we are able to change, to repair our worn-out parts and replace old cells with fresh new ones, then life and health continue.

The enemy of the body is not wear and tear. Our bodies are meant to be used—we cannot "save" ourselves by withdrawing from active life. The only mistake we can make is to fail to give the body the chance to repair itself, to replace worn-out material and make itself new again. We must provide our bodies with the right foods, and with the right rest, to enable it to care for itself as it has the innate capacity to do.

There are a number of experts in longevity who think that failure of the body to restore itself positively is the real culprit in aging, not time. They feel that if we could just continue to repair and transform our bodies, there would be no reason to die at any particular time. Certainly it is known that there are many little "deaths," small steps of decline that the body takes not because of age, but because some imbalance in the system prevents repair and renewal at some critical juncture. This would seem to indicate that a program which promotes a state of balanced health, which provides for proper food, exercise and rest, would be a step towards increased longevity.

I have designed the Body Type Diet with precisely these considerations in mind. It is for weight loss, and for beauty, but above all it is for improvement in the quality of life. My aim has always been to help you make the most of what you were born with, and to live all the potential that is yours. If your Body Type Diet becomes a means by which you enliven yourself to live life in all its fullness, then I have achieved my aim. Use it for good health and long life.

APPENDIX 1
RECIPES FOR GONADAL TYPES

STIR-FRIED CHICKEN

One whole chicken breast,
skinned and boned
1 cup fresh asparagus (if
available)

or 1 cup frozen asparagus,
thawed and cut into 1-inch
lengths
1 teaspoon vegetable oil

MARINADE: 2 teaspoons soy sauce
1 teaspoon corn starch
1 slice fresh ginger, minced (optional)
2 sliced green onions
1 teaspoon dry sherry (optional)

Cut boned chicken breast into ½-inch square pieces. Place in a bowl with the marinade. Heat ½ teaspoon oil in a wok or frying pan, add the vegetables and cook, stirring, 3–4 minutes or until just tender. Remove from the pan. Add the other ½ teaspoon of oil. Drain the marinade from the chicken and save it. Add the chicken to the hot oil and cook, stirring, about two minutes or until it turns white. Add vegetables and marinade and toss together 1 minute, until the sauce thickens and the vegetables are hot. Serves two.

SALMON STEAK FLORENTINE

2 4-ounce salmon steaks
1 bunch of fresh spinach
  (or use a package of frozen
  spinach)
½ teaspoon dried dill
  or 1 teaspoon of fresh, if
  available

1 lemon, cut into wedges
2 teaspoons vegetable oil
½ medium onion, chopped
⅛ teaspoon salt
Pinch of pepper

Wash the spinach carefully and shake off water. Cut into 1-inch strips. Wipe fish with a damp cloth and arrange in a single layer on a broiler pan. Broil about 4 inches from the heat for 5 minutes. Turn, sprinkle with salt and pepper, and brush the tops lightly with 1 teaspoon of oil. Sprinkle on the dill. Return to the broiler and broil 5 minutes more. Meanwhile, heat the remaining oil in a skillet. Cook onion until soft. Stir in the spinach, cover pan and cook, stirring occasionally, over high heat for 3 minutes, or until spinach is wilted and bright green. To serve, spoon spinach onto a warm platter and lay salmon steaks on top. Garnish with lemon wedges. Serves two.

MARINATED FISH WITH VEGETABLES

1½ pounds of white fish fillet
  such as flounder or sole
2 tablespoons lemon juice
½ large onion
2 small carrots
2 celery stalks
¼ cup of white wine vinegar

2 teaspoons of vegetable oil
2 teaspoons dried thyme
⅛ teaspoon of pepper
1 bay leaf
¾ teaspoon of salt
½ teaspoon of paprika
½ cup of water
Lettuce, parsley, lemon wedges

Wipe fish with a damp cloth and cut into serving-size pieces. Sprinkle with lemon juice and set aside. Julienne (cut into thin, 1-inch strips) the onion, celery and carrots into small strips. Combine vinegar, water, thyme, pepper, bay leaf and ½ teaspoon of salt. In a large skillet, heat oil and cook fish over medium heat for five minutes, then turn and cook 3–5 minutes more, or until fish flakes easily with a fork. Remove from the skillet and place in a shallow pan. In the same skillet, cook the carrots for two minutes. Add onion and celery and cook, stirring, two minutes more. Pour in vinegar mixture, cover and simmer 1 minute. Spoon vegetables and sauce over fish and let cool. Cover and refrigerate four hours or overnight. Serve cold fish on a lettuce-lined platter, garnished with parsley and lemon wedges. Serves six (a large recipe good for a party).

CHICKEN SALAD WITH YOGURT

2 whole chicken breasts
½ cup plain yogurt
1 green onion (optional)
½ teaspoon dried dill or
   1 teaspoon fresh dill

⅓ teaspoon salt
Lettuce leaves and tomato
   wedges

Cook chicken breasts in water to cover 25–30 minutes, until just tender. Cool in broth, remove fat, and save broth for another recipe. Remove the cooked chicken from the bone and cut into chunks. Mix with yogurt, salt, dill and green onion. Cover and chill. Serve on lettuce leaves garnished with tomato wedges. Serves four.

STIR-FRIED FISH FILLETS

½ pound of firm white fish fillets
1 teaspoon soy sauce
2 teaspoons water
2 teaspoons vegetable oil
1 bunch broccoli, cut into florets

½ teaspoon sesame oil (if
   available)
½ teaspoon corn starch
1 slice fresh ginger, minced

Heat 1 teaspoon of oil in a skillet or wok. Add the fish and ginger and cook, stirring very gently so that fish cooks evenly but does not come apart. When fish starts to turn white, remove from the pan. Pre-cook the broccoli by placing it in a small amount of boiling water for a few minutes. Drain. Heat the remaining teaspoon of oil in the skillet and add the broccoli, stir-frying 1–2 minutes until just crisp. Return fish to the pan, add the soy sauce, water and corn starch mixed together, and heat through so that sauce thickens and coats the fish and broccoli. At the last minute, sprinkle on the sesame oil. This is not necessary, but gives an interesting, Chinese taste. Serves four.

LEMON CHICKEN KABOBS

2 whole chicken breasts
2 teaspoons vegetable oil
2 small zucchini
½ teaspoon salt
Dash of cayenne pepper, if
    desired

1 large lemon
¼ pound fresh mushrooms
1 teaspoon cider vinegar

Grate 1 teaspoon of lemon peel from the lemon, then squeeze juice into a bowl. Add lemon peel, vinegar, salt and cayenne pepper. Bone and skin the chicken breasts and cut each breast into 4 or 5 roughly square pieces. Cut the zucchini into three pieces each. Add chicken, zucchini and mushrooms to the lemon juice mixture and toss lightly to coat each piece. Cover and refrigerate at least 3 hours, stirring occasionally. To cook, thread chicken, zucchini chunks and mushrooms alternately on 14-inch metal skewers. Place on a rack in the broiling pan, or over a barbecue, and broil 10–15 minutes, turning every few minutes. Brush several times with marinade mixture. Serves two.

EGGS MORNAY

2 soft-boiled eggs
1 teaspoon vegetable oil
¼ teaspoon dried basil
2 slices of whole-grain toast
2 medium ripe tomatoes, peeled
    and chopped

¼ teaspoon salt
2 slices of lowfat Swiss cheese
    (totalling 2 oz. cheese)

Make tomato sauce by cooking the garlic and basil in the oil for a minute or two. Add the tomatoes and salt and cook just until the tomatoes are heated through. In the meantime, soft-boil the eggs. Run them under cold water and peel them carefully. Wrap each egg in a slice of cheese. Divide the tomato sauce into two shallow baking dishes. Arrange an egg in the center of each. Broil about 5 minutes, until cheese is melted and slightly brown. Cut the toast into wedges and arrange around each dish. Serves two.

HERB OMELETTE

1 egg
1 tablespoon skim milk
2 teaspoons fresh herbs (basil,
    parsley, tarragon, thyme)

or 1 teaspoon dried herbs
1 teaspoon vegetable oil

Beat egg with milk in a bowl. Heat oil in a small skillet until hot, add egg and sprinkle with herbs. Lower the flame under the skillet and cook, drawing cooked egg away from the edges of the skillet with a spatula and letting the uncooked mixture run out toward the edges, until mixture is set. Fold in half and slide onto a plate. Serves one.

GREEK-STYLE EGGS

1 teaspoon olive or other
    vegetable oil
½ cup tomatoes
2 eggs, beaten

1 tablespoon Feta cheese
    (Ricotta cheese may be used
    if Feta is not available)

Cut up tomatoes into chunks and sautée in the oil 5–6 minutes. Add beaten eggs and Feta cheese and cook, stirring, until eggs are set and cheese is slightly melted. Serves one.

SPAGHETTI WITH CHEESE

2 ounces spaghetti, whole-wheat
    or spinach
4 ounces Parmesan cheese,
    grated

1 teaspoon butter

Bring water to a full boil in a large pot and add the spaghetti. Cook 7–9 minutes or until just tender but not soft. Drain. Add the butter and the cheese and return to the pot, tossing together over low heat until the cheese is melted and blended with the spaghetti. Serves one.

G-TYPE VEGETABLE SOUP

Zucchini
Beet tops
Romaine Lettuce

Watercress
Cucumber
Parsley

Cut the vegetables into chunks, using as much as you wish but approximately equal amounts of each. Use about ⅓ cup of each vegetable per serving. Place in a pot with water or chicken stock from which you have skimmed *all* fat. Cook for 5–10 minutes or until the vegetables are tender. You may eat as is or puree lightly in a blender if you prefer. A pinch of salt and pepper only is permitted. Eat as much as you wish while on your Last Five Pounds Diet—even between meals.

For convenience, you may prepare enough Vegetable Soup for several days. It keeps well in the refrigerator, and you can reheat it as needed.

CLEAR DIET DRESSING
FOR SALADS

The commercially-prepared diet salad dressings are acceptable provided you choose a clear one and not one of the creamy-looking ones such as roquefort. These may have fewer calories than *regular* creamy dressings, but are still too high in calories for your diet. If you want to make your dressing at home, use any of the following:

In a small saucepan combine 1 cup red wine vinegar and ½ cup chopped fresh herbs (try basil, parsley, tarragon, dill, thyme, or a combination). Bring to a boil. Cool and pour into a jar with a tight-fitting cover and let stand at room temperature for several days. Strain and use over any vegetable salad.
You can also mix 2 teaspoons of plain yogurt with a pinch of fresh or dried herbs and use it as a salad dressing.
Finally, fresh lemon juice squeezed over a salad is delicious.

PREPARING WHOLE GRAINS:
BULGHUR WHEAT, BROWN
RICE, AND MILLET

Whole grains are prepared in the same way as refined grains such as white rice, except that the cooking time is longer to allow the harder whole grains to be cooked through.
To prepare brown rice, placed washed rice in a saucepan with twice as much rice as water. Rice does not cook well in very small amounts, so it is a good idea to cook a minimum of ¾ cup rice at any one time, using 1½ cups water. Bring the water to a boil, lower heat and cover tightly. Allow to cook for about forty minutes, or until all the water is absorbed. Fluff with a fork and allow to stand for a few more minutes before serving.

To prepare millet and bulghur wheat, place in a pot with twice as much water as grain. Bring the water to a boil, cover and cook twenty minutes. For a richer flavor, use chicken stock instead of water.

APPENDIX 2

RECIPES FOR ADRENAL TYPES

STIR-FRIED FLANK STEAK

8 ounces of lean flank steak, sliced thinly on the diagonal
1 teaspoon vegetable oil

½ cup of bamboo shoots, sliced
1 cup of green peppers, sliced into strips

MARINADE: 2 teaspoons soy sauce
1 teaspoon corn starch
1 slice fresh ginger, minced (optional)
2 sliced green onions
1 teaspoon dry sherry (optional)

Place flank steak in a bowl with the marinade for 30 minutes before cooking. Heat ½ teaspoon oil in a wok or frying pan, add the vegetables and cook, stirring, 3–4 minutes or until just tender. Remove from the pan. Add the other ½ teaspoon of oil. Drain the marinade from the steak and save it. Add the steak to the hot oil and cook, stirring, about a minute or until it turns brown. Add vegetables and marinade and toss together 1 minute, until the sauce thickens and the vegetables are hot. Serves two.

CHICKEN VEGETABLE SOUP

1 whole chicken, cut up
3 celery ribs, cut into 1-inch pieces

1 box Matzoh-Ball and Soup Flavoring Mix
3 large carrots, cut into 1-inch pieces

Cover chicken pieces (except wings) and vegetables with water to cover in a large pot and cook 30 minutes or until chicken is tender.

Add soup seasoning mix to the pot. Meanwhile, prepare matzoh balls according to package directions, reducing oil to one tablespoon. Cook as directed. Chill soup in the refrigerator overnight, or until the fat is solid and easy to remove. Remove the skin from the chicken and all the fat from the soup. Serve as a family meal. Your portion is one piece of chicken, one matzoh ball and as many vegetables as you like. Serves six.

SOLE PROVENCAL

1 pound of sole (or you can use sea bass, flounder or other lean fish in season)
1 teaspoon of olive oil

4 fresh tomatoes, peeled and chopped, or 1 11-oz. can of whole tomatoes
1 clove of garlic (optional)
¼ pound mushrooms, sliced

Preheat the oven to 400 degrees. In a frying pan, cook mushrooms in the oil 2–3 minutes or until limp. Stir in the tomatoes and garlic and heat through. Add pepper to taste (no salt). Cut fish into four serving-sized pieces and place in a shallow baking dish. Cover with tomato-mushroom mixture. Bake uncovered, until fish flakes easily with a fork—about 10–15 minutes. Serves four.

RED SNAPPER "SCALLOPS"

8 ounces of red snapper, fresh or frozen
1 teaspoon vegetable oil
1 tablespoon dry white wine
1 tablespoon water

1 lime, cut into wedges
1 tablespoon cilantro ("Chinese parsley"), minced
or
1 tablespoon parsley, minced

Cut red snapper into "scallops"—approximately 1½ square-inch cubes. Heat the oil in a skillet and add fish. Sautée for 2 minutes, then add wine and water and cover. Cook about 10 minutes or until fish is opaque. Remove cover and squeeze ½ of the lime over the fish and sprinkle with the parsley or cilantro. Heat 1 minute more. Serve, garnished with the rest of the lime. Serves two.

CHICKEN BURGERS

2 whole chicken breasts, boned
    and skinned (turkey may be
    substituted)
2 tablespoons dried bread crumbs
½ medium onion, minced

4 large mushroom caps (optional)
1 egg
½ teaspoon salt
1 teaspoon of vegetable oil

Grind the chicken in a meat grinder or in a food processor (or buy ground chicken breast in the supermarket). Add the remaining ingredients except the mushrooms and oil. Blend and form into four patties. Heat the oil in a skillet and cook over medium heat, turning once. Meanwhile, place the mushrooms in a toaster oven or under the grill for 5 minutes. Serve the chickenburgers with a mushroom on each. Serves four.

TURKEY KABOBS

1 5–6 pound frozen turkey breast,
    thawed
¼ cup of soy sauce
¼ cup dry sherry
¼ cup Chinese plum sauce

1 tablespoon fresh ginger, minced
1 teaspoon salad oil
½ teaspoon crushed red pepper
1 bunch of green onions, sliced

Mix the soy sauce, sherry, ginger, oil, plum sauce and red pepper in a large bowl. Cut the turkey from the bone and cut into 2-inch cubes. Add to the marinade and toss to coat well. Cover and refrigerate for several hours or overnight. Thread the turkey cubes on metal skewers, alternating with onion pieces, and grill on a barbecue or in the oven for about 30 minutes, turning occasionally and brushing with marinade. Serves six.

CEVICHE WITH MELON

½ pound firm white fish
(flounder, sole, sea bass)—
very fresh
¼ medium red onion, sliced
1 whole clove

Juice of 1 lime
¼ teaspoon red pepper flakes
1 cup cantaloupe cubes
1 tablespoon chopped parsley

Combine fish in a small bowl with onion, lime juice, clove and red pepper. Refrigerate, covered, for six hours or overnight. The lime juice "cooks" the fish so that it is opaque rather than translucent. Just before serving, toss with the cantaloupe and parsley. Serves two.

EGGS MORNAY

2 soft-boiled eggs
1 teaspoon vegetable oil
¼ teaspoon dried basil
2 slices of toast

2 medium ripe tomatoes, peeled
2 slices of lowfat Swiss cheese

Make tomato sauce by cooking the garlic and basil in the oil for a minute or two. Add the tomatoes and cook just until the tomatoes are heated through. In the meantime, soft-boil the eggs. Run them under cold water and peel them carefully. Wrap each egg in a slice of cheese. Divide the tomato sauce into two shallow baking dishes. Arrange an egg in the center of each. Broil about 5 minutes, until cheese is melted and slightly brown. Cut the toast into wedges and arrange around each dish. Serves two.

A-TYPE VEGETABLE SOUP

Green Pepper
Zucchini
Celery

Chinese Peas (Snow Peas)
Tomato
Celery Tops

Use as many vegetables as you wish, but approximately equal quantities of all. About ⅓ cup of each vegetable should be used for each portion of soup. Chop the vegetables coarsely and place in a large pot with water or chicken broth from which you have removed *all* the fat. Bring to a boil and cook 5–10 minutes, or until vegetables are tender. You may add a pinch of pepper, but no salt. Eat as much of this soup as you want while on your Last Five Pounds Diet—even between meals if you wish.

For convenience, you may prepare several days worth of Vegetable Soup at once—it keeps well in the refrigerator and you need only reheat it as you wish.

PREPARING WHOLE GRAINS: BULGHUR WHEAT, BROWN RICE, AND MILLET

Whole grains are prepared in the same way as refined grains such as white rice, except that the cooking time is longer to allow the harder whole grains to be cooked through.

To prepare brown rice, place washed rice in a saucepan with twice as much rice as water. Rice does not cook well in very small amounts, so it is a good idea to cook a minimum of ¾ cup rice at any one time, using 1½ cups water. Bring the water to a boil, lower heat and cover tightly. Allow to cook for about forty minutes, or until all the water is absorbed. Fluff with a fork and allow to stand for a few more minutes before serving.

To prepare millet and bulghur wheat, place in a pot with twice as much water as grain. Bring the water to a boil, cover and cook twenty minutes. For a richer flavor, use chicken stock instead of water.

STIR-FRIED CHICKEN

One whole chicken breast, boned
   and skinned
½ cup green beans, sliced

1 teaspoon vegetable oil
½ cup celery, sliced

MARINADE: 2 teaspoons soy sauce
             1 teaspoon corn starch
             1 slice fresh ginger, minced (optional)
             2 sliced green onions
             1 teaspoon dry sherry (optional)

Cut boned chicken breast into ½-inch square pieces. Place in a bowl with the marinade. Heat ½ teaspoon oil in a wok or frying pan, add the vegetables and cook, stirring, 3–4 minutes or until just tender. Remove from the pan. Add the other ½ teaspoon of oil. Drain the marinade from the chicken and save it. Add the chicken to the hot oil and cook, stirring, about two minutes or until it turns white. Add vegetables and marinade and toss together 1 minute, until the sauce thickens and the vegetables are hot. Serves two.

SEAFOOD VERONIQUE

1 pound seafood (flounder,
   haddock, sole or other firm
   white fish—fresh or frozen)
1 egg
2 tablespoons chopped chives
3 tablespoons plain yogurt
½ pound seedless grapes

1 tablespoon grated Parmesan
   cheese
1 tablespoon diet mayonnaise
½ clove garlic, crushed (optional)
2 tablespoons of lemon juice
1 lemon, cut into wedges

Slightly beat the egg, then blend in the plain yogurt, chives, diet mayonnaise, and a sliver of the garlic. Cut fish into 1-inch chunks and combine in a bowl with the lemon juice and the rest of the garlic. Add the grapes and toss together to combine. Preheat oven to 400 degrees. Spoon the fish and grapes into four individual baking dishes or one 8-inch square dish. Spoon plain yogurt mixture over fish and top with grated cheese. Bake 12–15 minutes, until top is hot and bubbly. Garnish with lemon wedges. Serves four.

CHICKEN BREAST PIQUANT

1 whole chicken breast, skin
   removed
1 teaspoon vegetable oil
½ clove garlic, chopped
   (optional)
1 ripe tomato, coarsely chopped

1 small can water-packed
   artichoke hearts
1 teaspoon tomato paste
1 tablespoon wine vinegar
½ teaspoon dried thyme

Heat the vegetable oil in a frying pan and brown the chicken five minutes on each side. Remove it from the pan and add all the remaining ingredients except the artichoke hearts. Stir and heat to boiling. Return the chicken to the pan, cover and cook over low heat 20–25 minutes or until chicken is tender. Add the artichoke hearts for the last five minutes and allow to heat through.

FRUIT ICE

1 pound of ripe fruit
   (strawberries, mango,
   papaya, peaches—you
   choose)

⅛ cup sugar
1 envelope unflavored gelatin
¼ cup lemon juice

Sprinkle gelatin over lemon juice, let stand. In a small pan, combine sugar with 1 cup of water. Stir over low heat until sugar dissolves; bring to boil and boil gently, uncovered and without stirring, five minutes. Remove from heat. Add the gelatin and stir until dissolved. Puree the fruit in a blender until smooth, and add gelatin mixture to it; blend until smooth. Turn into a 8 x 8 x 2″ pan. Freeze about 2 hours. Turn into a chilled bowl and beat quickly with a mixer or rotary beater until smooth but not melted. Return to the pan and freeze several hours, until firm. Serves eight.

CHOCOLATE COOKIES

3 egg whites, at room
   temperature
6 squares of unsweetened
   chocolate, melted and cooled

½ teaspoon of vanilla extract
½ cup of sugar

Preheat oven to 350 degrees. Grease 2 cookie sheets. In a small mixer bowl, beat egg whites until stiff. Add sugar, 1 tablespoon at a time, and continue beating until mixture is smooth and glossy and sugar is completely dissolved. Fold in chocolate and vanilla. Drop by teaspoonfuls onto the cookie sheets. Bake 15 minutes. Makes 60 cookies.

CLEAR DIET DRESSING
FOR SALADS

The commercially-prepared diet salad dressings are acceptable provided you choose a clear one and not one of the creamy-looking ones such as roquefort. These may have fewer calories than *regular* creamy dressings, but are still too high in calories for your diet. If you want to make your dressing at home, use any of the following:

In a small saucepan combine 1 cup red wine vinegar and ½ cup chopped fresh herbs (try basil, parsley, tarragon, dill, thyme, or a combination). Bring to a boil. Cool and pour into a jar with a tight-fitting cover and let stand at room temperature for several days. Strain and use over any vegetable salad.

A variation is to omit herbs from the preceding recipe and add 4 crushed cloves of garlic.

You can also mix 2 teaspoons of plain yogurt with a pinch of fresh or dried herbs and use it as a salad dressing.

Finally, fresh lemon juice squeezed over a salad is delicious.

APPENDIX 3
RECIPES FOR THYROID TYPES

MEXICAN STUFFED CHICKEN

2 chicken breasts, skinned and
   boned
1 tablespoon dried bread crumbs
1 tablespoon grated Parmesan
   cheese
2 tablespoons mild green chilis,
   chopped

½ teaspoon chili powder
1 egg, beaten
1 ounce Monterey Jack cheese,
   cut into two slices, 3-inches
   by 1-inch

Preheat oven to 375°. With a kitchen hammer or the side of a cleaver, pound out the boned breasts to ¼-inch thick. On each one, place a tablespoon of the chilis and a Monterey Jack cheese slice. Roll up and place, seam side down, in a baking dish. Brush with beaten egg. Mix together the bread crumbs, Parmesan cheese and chili powder and sprinkle over the chicken rolls, patting into place to form a crust. Bake for about 20 minutes— cheese inside will be melted and the crust nicely browned. Serves two.

STIR-FRIED CHICKEN

One whole chicken breast,   1 teaspoon vegetable oil
   skinned and boned.   1 cup green pepper, sliced
½ cup celery, sliced
MARINADE: 2 teaspoons soy sauce
          1 teaspoon corn starch
          1 slice fresh ginger, minced (optional)
          2 sliced green onions
          1 teaspoon dry sherry (optional)

Cut boned chicken breast into ½-inch square pieces. Place in a
bowl with the marinade. Heat ½ teaspoon oil in a wok or frying
pan, add the vegetables and cook, stirring, 3–4 minutes or until
just tender. Remove from the pan. Add the other ½ teaspoon of
oil. Drain the marinade from the chicken and save it. Add the
chicken to the hot oil and cook, stirring, about two minutes or
until it turns white. Add vegetables and marinade and toss together 1 minute, until the sauce thickens and the vegetables are
hot. Serves two.

SALMON STEAK
FLORENTINE

2 4-ounce salmon steaks   1 lemon, cut into wedges
1 bunch of fresh spinach   2 teaspoons vegetable oil
   (or use a package of frozen   ½ medium onion, chopped
   spinach)   ⅛ teaspoon salt
½ clove of garlic, crushed   Pinch of pepper
   (optional)
½ teaspoon dried dill
   or 1 teaspoon of fresh, if
   available

Wash the spinach carefully and shake off water. Cut into 1-inch
strips. Wipe fish with a damp cloth and arrange in a single layer
on a broiler pan. Broil about 4 inches from the heat for 5 minutes.
Turn, sprinkle with salt and pepper, and brush the tops lightly
with 1 teaspoon of oil. Sprinkle on the dill. Return to the broiler

and broil 5 minutes more. Meanwhile, heat the remaining oil in a skillet. Cook onion and garlic until soft. Stir in the spinach, cover pan and cook, stirring occasionally, over high heat for 3 minutes, or until spinach is wilted and bright green. To serve, spoon spinach onto a warm platter and lay salmon steaks on top. Garnish with lemon wedges. Serves two.

BARBECUED TUNA

½ pounds of fresh or frozen tuna
  (Albacore, if available)
2 ounces of frozen grapefruit
  juice
2 teaspoons lime juice
  (use lemon juice if lime is not
  available)

¼ teaspoon salt
¼ teaspoon Tabasco sauce
¼ teaspoon dried thyme
¼ teaspoon mustard

Combine grapefruit concentrate, lime or lemon juice, salt, mustard, thyme and Tabasco sauce in a bowl. Marinate fish for 30 minutes. Cook over barbecue grill, or in the oven broiler, for 15 minutes, turning several times and basting with marinade mixture. Fish is done when it flakes easily with a fork. Garnish with a sprinkling of paprika. Serves two.

CHEF'S SALAD

2 ounces cold cooked chicken
Lettuce, tomato, cucumber,
  celery, sprouts, as much as
  you like
2 teaspoons of any clear (not
  creamy) diet dressing

2 ounces hard cheese
  (Parmesan or Romano)

Slice chicken and vegetables, toss together with dressing, and serve. Serves one.

SESAME SHRIMP WITH ASPARAGUS

4 ounces of shrimp
1 bunch of asparagus, sliced into
    1-inch pieces
1 teaspoon soy sauce
1 teaspoon vegetable oil

1 small slice of fresh ginger,
    minced (optional)
2 teaspoons sesame seeds
½ teaspoon corn starch

Peel shrimp and make a cut up the back, removing the black vein along the back. Place the sesame seeds in a wok or frying pan without oil and toast 2–3 minutes, watching to see they do not burn. Remove from pan. Heat ½ teaspoon of oil in the pan and cook the asparagus 2 minutes, until not quite done. Remove asparagus from the pan. Heat the remaining ½ teaspoon of oil and cook the shrimp 3–4 minutes, until they turn pink. Add asparagus and cook ½ minute longer. Stir together soy sauce, ginger, and corn starch and add to the pan, stirring to coat shrimp and asparagus. Sprinkle with toasted sesame seeds. Serves one.

HERB OMELETTE

2 eggs
1 tablespoon skim milk
2 teaspoons fresh herbs (basil,
    parsley, tarragon, thyme)
    or 1 teaspoon dried herbs

1 teaspoon vegetable oil

Beat eggs with milk in a bowl. Heat oil in a small skillet until hot, add eggs and sprinkle with herbs. Lower the flame under the skillet and cook, drawing cooked eggs away from the edges of the skillet with a spatula and letting the uncooked mixture run out toward the edges, until mixture is set. Fold in half and slide onto a plate. Serves one.

T-TYPE VEGETABLE SOUP

Green beans   Yellow squash or zucchini
Celery   Celery tops
Carrots   Carrot tops

Cut the vegetables into chunks, using as much as you wish but approximately equal amounts of each. Use about ⅓ cup of each vegetable per serving. Place in a pot with water or chicken stock from which you have skimmed *all* fat. Cook for 5–10 minutes or until the vegetables are tender. You may eat as is or puree lightly in a blender if you prefer. A pinch of salt and pepper only is permitted. Eat as much as you wish while on your Last Five Pounds Diet—even between meals.

For convenience you may prepare enough of your Vegetable Soup for several days. It keeps well in the refrigerator, and you can reheat it as you need it.

CHICKEN STEW

2 whole chicken breasts   1 teaspoon curry powder
2 cups water   ¼ teaspoon dried thyme
1 celery rib, cut into 2-inch   Dash cayenne pepper
  pieces   ¼ medium onion
½ teaspoon salt   ½ green pepper, diced
½ pound zucchini   1 teaspoon vegetable oil
½ clove garlic, crushed   ½ bay leaf
1 14-oz. can tomatoes, with juice

Place chicken in a medium pan with water, bay leaf, celery and ½ teaspoon salt. Bring to a boil, reduce heat and simmer 30 minutes, or until chicken is tender. Cool chicken in broth in the refrigerator overnight, or until fat is fully solid. Remove every trace of fat. Cut up chicken into bite-sized pieces, discarding the skin. Save 1 cup of broth. In the same pot, saute onion, peppers, garlic and seasonings in the oil for a few minutes. Add tomatoes, zucchini and broth and simmer 5 minutes, until zucchini is tender. Add chicken and heat through. Serves four.

CHICKEN BREAST PIQUANT

1 whole chicken breast, skin
   removed
1 teaspoon vegetable oil
½ clove garlic, chopped
   (optional)
1 ripe tomato, coarsely chopped

1 small can water-packed
   artichoke hearts
1 teaspoon tomato paste
1 tablespoon wine vinegar
¼ teaspoon salt
½ teaspoon dried thyme

Sprinkle the chicken breast lightly with salt. Heat the vegetable oil in a frying pan and brown the chicken five minutes on each side. Remove it from the pan and add all the remaining ingredients except the artichoke hearts. Stir and heat to boiling. Return the chicken to the pan, cover and cook over low heat 20–25 minutes or until chicken is tender. Add the artichoke hearts for the last five minutes and allow to heat through.

BAKED HALIBUT STEAK

2 fresh or frozen halibut steaks,
   4 ounces each
⅛ teaspoon of paprika
3 teaspoons lemon juice

¼ teaspoon salt
Dash pepper
2 green onions, sliced
½ teaspoon vegetable oil

Thaw fish steaks, if frozen. Sprinkle with lemon juice, salt, paprika and pepper. Place in a shallow baking dish and let stand to marinate for 30 minutes. Cook the onions for 2 minutes in the oil, then spoon over fish. Bake, covered, 15–20 minutes in a 350-degree oven. Remove cover for last three minutes to allow onions to brown. Serves two.

PREPARING WHOLE GRAINS: BULGHUR WHEAT, BROWN RICE, AND MILLET

Whole grains are prepared in the same way as refined grains such as white rice, except that the cooking time is longer to allow the harder whole grains to be cooked through.

To prepare brown rice, place washed rice in a saucepan with twice as much rice as water. Rice does not cook well in very small amounts, so it is a good idea to cook a minimum of ¾ cup rice at any one time, using 1½ cups water. Bring the water to a boil, lower heat and cover tightly. Allow to cook for about forty minutes, or until all the water is absorbed. Fluff with a fork and allow to stand for a few more minutes before serving.

To prepare millet and bulghur wheat, place in a pot with twice as much water as grain. Bring the water to a boil, cover and cook twenty minutes. For a richer flavor, use chicken stock instead of water.

TURKEY KABOBS

5–6 pounds frozen turkey breast, thawed
½ cup of soy sauce
¼ cup dry sherry
1 tablespoon fresh ginger, minced
1 teaspoon salad oil
½ teaspoon crushed red pepper
1 bunch of green onions, sliced

Mix the soy sauce, sherry, ginger, oil and red pepper in a large bowl. Cut the turkey from the bone and cut into 2-inch cubes. Add to the marinade and toss to coat well. Cover and refrigerate for several hours or overnight. Thread the turkey cubes on metal skewers, alternating with onion pieces, and grill on a barbecue or in the oven for about 30 minutes, turning occasionally and brushing with marinade. Serves six.

CLEAR DIET DRESSING
FOR SALADS

The commercially-prepared diet salad dressings are acceptable provided you choose a clear one and not one of the creamy-looking ones such as roquefort. These may have fewer calories than *regular* creamy dressings, but are still too high in calories for your diet. If you want to make your dressing at home, use any of the following:

In a small saucepan combine 1 cup red wine vinegar and ½ cup chopped fresh herbs (try basil, parsley, tarragon, dill, thyme, or a combination). Bring to a boil. Cool and pour into a jar with a tight-fitting cover and let stand at room temperature for several days. Strain and use over any vegetable salad.

A variation is to omit herbs from the preceding recipe and add 4 crushed cloves of garlic.

You can also mix 2 teaspoons of plain yogurt with a pinch of fresh or dried herbs and use it as a salad dressing.

Finally, fresh lemon juice squeezed over a salad is delicious.

APPENDIX 4
RECIPES FOR PITUITARY TYPES

PREPARING ORGAN MEATS:
LIVER, KIDNEYS, AND
HEART

All organ meats—liver, kidneys, and heart—are highly perishable. Buy only what you will be eating within the next two or three days at the most.

Liver: To prepare any kind of liver—beef, calf or chicken—wipe it first with a damp cloth, then remove the thin outer skin and veining. The cooking method is the same for all types. To grill, place it 3–4 inches away from the heat source. Cook only long enough to cook through—about a minute on each side. Cooking too long, or too close to the heat, will toughen liver. The center should remain just slightly pink. Liver can also be sauteed in a frying pan in a teaspoon of vegetable oil.

Kidneys: Veal Kidneys are surprisingly tasty; the English eat them for breakfast all the time. To prepare, wipe the kidney with a damp cloth, then split them and remove the cores. The white membranes should be snipped away. Cut them in half and expose the cut side to the heat first. They may be panfried in a teaspoon of vegetable oil, or broiled in the oven. Cook them until the center is just slightly pink—about 5 minutes on each side.

Heart: Heart is a muscle, rather than a *true* organ meat, and tends to be somewhat tough. It is best prepared ground. Ask your butcher to do this for you, or put it through a meat grinder or food processor. Form into a patty and sautee in 1 teaspoon of vegetable oil, or broil in the oven, until meat is no longer pink, about 25–30 minutes.

BROILED SHRIMP WITH
LEMON

Peel the shrimp and, with a sharp knife, make a shallow cut along the back and remove the vein (actually the intestine). Sprinkle with lemon juice and a small amount of salt. Place the shrimp under the broiler about 3 inches from the heat. Broil 3 minutes, turn and broil three minutes more. Do not overcook—shrimp should be cooked just until the flesh is opaque. Serve with more lemon juice if desired.

STIR-FRIED CHICKEN

One whole chicken breast, boned   1 teaspoon vegetable oil
    and skinned   ½ cup mushrooms, sliced
½ cup zucchini, sliced

MARINADE: 2 teaspoons soy sauce
          1 teaspoon corn starch
          1 slice fresh ginger, minced (optional)
          2 sliced green onions
          1 teaspoon dry sherry (optional)

Cut boned chicken breast into ½-inch square pieces. Place in a bowl with the marinade. Heat ½ teaspoon oil in a wok or frying pan, add the vegetables and cook, stirring, 3–4 minutes or until just tender. Remove from the pan. Add the other ½ teaspoon of oil. Drain the marinade from the chicken and save it. Add the chicken to the hot oil and cook, stirring, about two minutes or until it turns white. Add vegetables and marinade and toss together 1 minute, until the sauce thickens and the vegetables are hot. Serves two.

CHICKEN BREAST

2 whole chicken breasts, skin removed
1 teaspoon vegetable oil
½ clove garlic, chopped
1 ripe tomato, coarsely chopped

1 small can water-packed artichoke hearts
1 teaspoon tomato paste
1 tablespoon wine vinegar
¼ teaspoon salt
½ teaspoon dried thyme

Sprinkle the chicken breast lightly with salt. Heat the vegetable oil in a frying pan and brown the chicken five minutes on each side. Remove it from the pan and add all the remaining ingredients except the artichoke hearts. Stir and heat to boiling. Return the chicken to the pan, cover and cook over low heat 20–25 minutes or until chicken is tender. Add the artichoke hearts for the last five minutes and allow to heat through. Serves four.

LEMON CHICKEN KABOBS WITH MUSHROOMS AND ZUCCHINI

1 chicken breast, skinned
1 lemon
1 teaspoon vegetable oil
2 small zucchini
1 teaspoon vinegar

½ clove garlic
⅛ teaspoon cayenne pepper
¼ pound mushrooms
¼ teaspoon salt

Three hours before serving, marinate the chicken as follows: grate 1 teaspoon lemon peel from the lemon, then squeeze juice into a bowl. Add lemon peel, oil, vinegar, salt, cayenne and garlic. Cut the chicken into four or five roughly square pieces. Cut the zucchini into 3 pieces each. Add chicken, trimmed mushrooms and zucchini pieces to the marinade and toss to coat each piece. Refrigerate. To cook, thread chicken pieces, zucchini chunks and mushrooms alternately on 14-inch skewers. Place skewers on a rack in the broiling pan, or over a barbecue, and broil 10–15 minutes, turning occasionally. Brush with marinade mixture when you turn. Serves two.

ONION-CELERY OMELETTE

2 eggs   ½ cup sliced celery
1 teaspoon water   2 sliced green onions
2 teaspoons vegetable oil

Heat 1 teaspoon vegetable oil in a small frying pan. Sautee celery and onions 4–5 minutes, until tender. Remove from the pan. Beat the eggs together with the water until mixed. Heat remaining oil in the pan and add the eggs. Gently stir the eggs in the pan and tip the egg mixture towards the edge of the pan until set. Put the celery-onion mixture on one side of the eggs, fold the egg mixture in half over the filling, and slide onto a plate. Serves one.

STIR-FRIED GREEN BEANS

1 cup of green beans   1 teaspoon vegetable oil
⅛ teaspoon salt

Slice beans crosswise into 1-inch pieces. Heat the oil in a frying pan and add beans. Cook, stirring, 3–5 minutes or just until beans are tender. Sprinkle with salt and serve.

POACHED PEAR

Bring 2 cups of water to a boil and add 1 clove and 1 stick of cinnamon. Reduce heat. Simmer pear gently in the spiced water until tender—about 15–20 minutes.

SOLE PROVENCAL

1 pound of sole (or you can use   4 fresh tomatoes, peeled and
    sea bass, flounder or other   chopped, or 1 11-oz. can of
    lean fish in season)   whole tomatoes
1 teaspoon olive oil   1 clove garlic, crushed
                                    ¼ pound mushrooms, sliced

Preheat the oven to 400 degrees. In a frying pan, cook mushrooms in the oil 2–3 minutes or until limp. Stir in the tomatoes and garlic and heat through. Add pepper to taste (no salt). Cut fish into four serving-sized pieces and place in a shallow baking dish. Cover with tomato-mushroom mixture. Bake, uncovered, until fish flakes easily with a fork—about 10–15 minutes. Serves four.

STIR-FRIED FISH FILLETS

½ pound firm white fish fillets
½ cup mushrooms
1 teaspoon soy sauce
2 teaspoons water

2 teaspoons vegetable oil
1 cup green beans
½ teaspoon sesame oil (if
    available)
½ teaspoon corn starch
1 slice fresh ginger, minced

Heat 1 teaspoon of oil in a skillet or wok. Add the fish and ginger and cook, stirring very gently so that fish cooks evenly but does not come apart. When fish starts to turn white, remove from the pan. Heat the remaining teaspoon of oil in the skillet and add the green beans. Stir-frying 3–4 minutes until just crisp, add the mushrooms and stir-fry 1 minute more. Return fish to the pan, add the soy sauce, water and corn starch mixed together, and heat through so that sauce thickens and coats the fish and vegetables. At the last moment, sprinkle on the sesame oil. This is not necessary, but gives an interesting, Chinese taste. Serves four.

BAKED SESAME FISH

2 frozen fish steaks about 1-inch
    thick, 4 ounces each (cod,
    whitefish or other firm fish)
    or 2 fresh fish pieces, cut

into 4 ounce steaks, 1-inch
    thick
2 tablespoons sesame seeds
1 egg, beaten

Preheat oven to 350°. Brush fish on top with beaten egg and press sesame seeds firmly onto the surface to form a "crust." (You will not need all the egg, so save for scrambled eggs at another meal). Place fish in a small baking dish and bake about 20 minutes, or until sesame seeds are browned and fish flakes easily when prodded with a fork. Serves two.

CRACKED CRABS P-TYPE

4 whole cleaned crabs in their   ½ lemon, cut into wedges
   shells   Dashes of salt and pepper
½ lemon, sliced

Crab is so delicious by itself it needs no special preparation to make it enjoyable. Simply bring to a boil a large pot of water. Drop in the crabs and lemon slices and boil 15–20 minutes. Drain, crack shells with a hammer and serve with lemon wedges, salt and pepper. Crabs can also be bought in many fish markets already cooked. Serves two.

P-TYPE VEGETABLE SOUP

Beets   Beet tops
Okra   Mushrooms
Green beans   Zucchini
Celery   Green onions

Use as much vegetable as you wish, but approximately equal amounts of each. Use about ⅓ cup of each vegetable for each serving. Chop the vegetables and place them in a pot with water, or with beef or chicken stock from which you have removed every trace of fat. Bring to a boil and cook 5 minutes, or until vegetables are just tender. You may then puree the soup in a blender or eat as is. You may add just a pinch of salt and pepper. Eat as much of this soup as you wish when you are on the Last Five Pounds Diet, even between meals. For convenience you may prepare enough of your Vegetable Soup to last for several days. It keeps well in the refrigerator, and you can simply reheat it as needed.

BAKED HALIBUT STEAK

2 fresh or frozen halibut steaks, 4 ounces each
⅛ teaspoon paprika
3 teaspoons lemon juice
¼ teaspoon salt
Dash pepper
2 green onions, sliced
½ teaspoon vegetable oil

Thaw fish steaks, if frozen. Sprinkle with lemon juice, salt, paprika and pepper. Place in a shallow baking dish and let stand to marinate for 30 minutes. Cook the onions for 2 minutes in the oil, then spoon over fish. Bake, covered, 15–20 minutes in a 350-degree oven. Remove cover for last three minutes to allow onions to brown. Serves two.

MARINATED FISH WITH VEGETABLES

(A larger recipe, good for a summer party)
1½ pounds white fish fillet such as flounder or sole
2 tablespoons lemon juice
½ large onion
2 small carrots
2 celery stalks
¼ cup white wine vinegar
½ clove garlic, crushed (optional)
2 teaspoons vegetable oil
2 teaspoons dried thyme
⅛ teaspoon pepper
1 bay leaf
¾ teaspoon salt
½ teaspoon paprika
½ cup water
Lettuce, parsley, lemon wedges

Wipe fish with a damp cloth and cut into serving-size pieces. Sprinkle with lemon juice and set aside. Cut onion, celery and carrots into small strips. Combine vinegar, water, thyme, pepper, bay leaf and ½ teaspoon of salt. In a large skillet, heat oil and cook fish over medium heat for five minutes, then turn and cook 3–5 minutes more, or until fish flakes easily with a fork. Remove from the skillet and place in a shallow pan. In the same skillet, cook the carrots for two minutes. Add onion, celery and garlic and cook, stirring, two minutes more. Pour in vinegar mixture, cover and simmer 1 minute. Spoon vegetables and sauce over fish and let cool. Cover and refrigerate four hours or overnight. Serve cold fish on a lettuce-lined platter, garnished with parsley and lemon wedges. Serves six.

SALMON STEAK
FLORENTINE

2 4-ounce salmon steaks
1 bunch fresh spinach (or use a
    package of frozen spinach)
½ clove garlic, crushed (optional)
½ teaspoon dried dill or 1
    teaspoon fresh, if available

2 teaspoons vegetable oil
½ medium onion, chopped
⅛ teaspoon salt
Pinch of pepper

Wash the spinach carefully and shake off water. Cut into 1-inch strips. Wipe fish with a damp cloth and arrange in a single layer on a broiler pan. Broil about 4 inches from the heat for 5 minutes. Turn, sprinkle with salt and pepper, and brush the tops lightly with 1 teaspoon of oil. Sprinkle on the dill. Return to the broiler and broil 5 minutes more. Meanwhile, heat the remaining oil in a skillet. Cook onion and garlic until soft. Stir in the spinach, cover pan and cook, stirring occasionally, over high heat for 3 minutes, or until spinach is wilted and bright green. To serve, spoon spinach onto a warm platter and lay salmon steaks on top. Garnish with lemon wedges. Serves two.

CLEAR DIET DRESSING
FOR SALADS

The commercially-prepared diet salad dressings are acceptable provided you choose a clear one and not one of the creamy-looking ones such as roquefort. These may have fewer calories than *regular* creamy dressings, but are still too high in calories for your diet. If you want to make your dressing at home, use any of the following:

In a small saucepan combine 1 cup red wine vinegar and ½ cup chopped fresh herbs (try basil, parsley, tarragon, dill, thyme, or a combination). Bring to a boil. Cool and pour into a jar with a tight-fitting cover and let stand at room temperature for several days. Strain and use over any vegetable salad.

A variation is to omit herbs from the preceding recipe and add 4 crushed cloves of garlic.

Finally, fresh lemon juice squeezed over a salad is delicious.

PREPARING WHOLE GRAINS: BULGHUR WHEAT, BROWN RICE, AND MILLET

Whole grains are prepared in the same way as refined grains such as white rice, except that the cooking time is longer to allow the harder whole grains to be cooked through.

To prepare brown rice, place washed rice in a saucepan with twice as much rice as water. Rice does not cook well in very small amounts, so it is a good idea to cook a minimum of ¾ cup rice at any one time, using 1½ cups water. Bring the water to a boil, lower heat and cover tightly. Allow to cook for about forty minutes, or until all the water is absorbed. Fluff with a fork and allow to stand for a few more minutes before serving.

To prepare millet and bulghur wheat, place in a pot with twice as much water as grain. Bring the water to a boil, cover and cook twenty minutes. For a richer flavor, use chicken stock instead of water.

INDEX